Conceive

THE MERCIER APPROACH

To Sabra
Thank you for
your support

JENNIFER D. MERCIER

Published by Known Publishing, 2021

Full colour print: 978-1-913717-61-2

Conceive B&W: 978-1-913717-57-5

Ebook: 978-1-913717-58-2

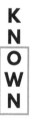

www.get-known.co.uk

"We come into this world through women who are told to be afraid of their birthing bodies while they drink Coke and eat McDonald's and fathers whose sperm marinated in trans-generationally disruptive pesticides. We are ultrasounded in the womb regularly, birthed surgically, formula-fed, vaccinated, left by mothers who have a three-week maternity leave, schooled into a state of near irreversible brain-washing while being microwaved by 5G networks. As adults, we work jobs that mean nothing and take everything and engage in relationships that could never possibly heal all of the unexamined wounds we bring to them, all while swimming in a bath of chemicals."

– KELLY BROGAN, MD

OWN YOURSELF

"The waiting time in between cycles and tests and procedures is probably the most challenging period of the fertility process. For every day that I was not fully engaged with injections or ultrasounds or paperwork, I had time to question what we were doing and why we were doing it."

– MIRIAM ZOLL

CRACKED OPEN: LIBERTY, FERTILITY AND THE HIGH PURSUIT OF HIGH-TECH BABIES

Dedication

I'd like to dedicate Conceive to my children, Clair and Seth. For without them my work would be dull and I wouldn't have such a fruitful personal fertility story to share. God's grace in this writing is visible throughout each page and I am thankful.

The Butterfly Struggle

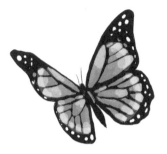

A man found a cocoon of a butterfly. One day a small opening appeared. He sat and watched the butterfly for several hours as it struggled to squeeze its body through the tiny hole. Then it stopped, as if it couldn't go further.

So the man decided to help the butterfly. He took a pair of scissors and snipped off the remaining bits of cocoon. The butterfly emerged easily but it had a swollen body and shriveled wings.

The man continued to watch it, expecting that any minute the wings would enlarge and expand enough to support the body. Neither happened! In fact, the butterfly spent the rest of its life crawling around. It was never able to fly.

What the man in his kindness and haste did not understand: the restricting cocoon and the struggle required by the butterfly to get through the opening was a way of forcing the fluid from the body into the wings so that it would be ready for flight once that was achieved.

Sometimes struggles are exactly what we need in our lives. Going through life with no obstacles would cripple us. We will not be as strong as we could have been and we would never fly.

"The art of medicine consists of amusing the patient while nature cures the disease. Doctors put drugs of which they know very little into bodies of which they know less for diseases of which they know nothing at all."

VOLTAIRE

Contents

Introduction

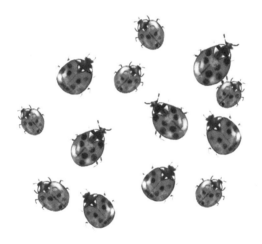

H ave you ever heard the story about the little girl who wandered around in search of ladybugs? She turns over rocks, runs through fields grabbing fistfuls of leaves, plays in the creek, but the poor girl has little luck. She only finds a few and feels like giving up. Now, it's late afternoon, the sun is hot overhead, she's tired, discouraged, and decides to take a nap in the soft green grass. Funny thing is, she wakes and there are ladybugs crawling all over her! Sometimes, gently laying down the reigns and taking a rest can produce the best results.

This is exactly what I offer with Merciér Therapy.

The majority of women who want to become pregnant will stop at nothing short of hitting the proverbial brick wall, thinking they're going to punch through this wall, only to end up smashing their bodies and hearts against those bricks over and over again. Eventually the emotional, physical, and mental exhaustion can be devastating and probably will end up causing overall endocrine disruption which can lead to adrenal dysfunction, among other things. Aside from maybe not solving the problem, this in and of itself can be a challenge to getting back to a state of wellness. The cascade of events can leave one feeling overwhelmed, defeated, deflated, depressed, and full to the brim with anxiety.

In over twenty years of practice, I've seen and heard a variety of stories from women. Some are wonderful and others not-so-wonderful. My work has blessed me in ways that are indescribable. Because of Merciér Therapy I have two amazing children and many, many other women have had babies with little to no intervention. Women have flown in from all over the world seeking Merciér Therapy and have had great successes.

Like Saoirse and Conor Walsh, a wonderful couple whose story unfortunately sounds very familiar to many of my patients:

"Before I started seeing Dr. Jennifer Merciér, I was in the cycle of belief that only medicine would get me pregnant. No one could tell me otherwise. After three failed Clomid and three failed fresh IVF and two FET cycles I realized that I was spinning my wheels. I was told at age 32 that I would not conceive without IVF.

I was told that my conception needed to be forced. I was told that my chances of conceiving naturally were slim to nothing. Endometriosis was governing my pelvis and causing me tremendous pain. My menstrual cycles were very heavy with a lot of cramping. Both tubes are open and still I was given a dismal conclusion. My clinic made me feel as though they would get me pregnant with little to no effort and it would not be a big deal.

"It turned into a circus for me.

"I followed the instructions from the clinic. I was obedient to the schedule. I stimulated well with all six cycles. The scenario always looked promising. I was always reassured that the follicles were growing and retrieved matching the plan. My embryos, according to the embryologist, were perfect. With each transfer came promise and hope.

"My pregnancy tests were always negative. It was such a low blow. I did what I was told. I followed the rules. In the end, my husband and I were left 31,000.00 € (Euros)($34,000.00) in debt. No more embryos and marital trauma.

"We felt broken, so we took a vacation from our home in Ireland and flew over to meet with Dr. Jennifer Merciér. We decided long ago that if we did not become pregnant with our current plan then I would try the Shared Journey Fertility program. However, there was no one in Ireland practicing. We could have gone to the UK but decided to make the trip to work with Jennifer. I had heard many podcast interviews of Jennifer speaking about her own struggles with endometriosis and felt a sense of connection. Upon arrival we immediately felt a warm welcome in Saint Charles, Illinois. Sleepy from jetlag, we ventured to Dr. Merciér's office the following day. We had the pleasure of meeting and spending time with her as she carefully took my history. The three of us reviewed all the tests, surgical report, and labs. After learning that I had a great egg reserve, slightly low thyroid, and some surgical scar tissue we proceeded into the Merciér Therapy sessions. I had a 90-minute session each day for four consecutive days. I was SORE. This was not what I had expected! I don't know what I expected but it wasn't this. It was the deepest pelvic work I'd ever experienced done on my abdomen, but almost immediately my endometriosis pain was near obsolete! Prior to the work, I had a stabbing pain in my rectum upon sitting. This was a constant. Now it is no more.

"After the fourth day we talked about how to proceed. She carefully explained that she wanted me to monitor my cycles and gave me a journal in which to track ovulation. I had never been taught about cervical fluid changes or LH surge. I was astounded at what I had observed for years but never knew the purpose.

"Suddenly, I felt in charge of my own cycles. This really empowered me to be my best from a nutrition and exercise standpoint. It changed my entire perspective from hopeless to hopeful.[1]

"I noticed that the two cycles that I monitored were consistently showing me that I was ovulating. Then my third cycle never started because I was pregnant! I could not believe my eyes. After everything I'd gone through and here I was with a positive home pregnancy test! Pure magic. My husband was elated. My pregnancy was uneventful, and I gave birth with a midwife to our daughter in May 2019. I now reflect back on all of the medical interventions, each time I was told that I would not get pregnant without IVF, all of the failed cycles, all of the time spent for each appointment, exam and procedure, and thousands of euros spent to bring us no closer to our hope of building our family. I really enjoyed my time with Dr. Jenny. She encouraged us and instilled a level of hope that we thought was gone forever. She did not promise us anything except for her help and dedication. She said that she would walk with us down the path. She did exactly that. She did not speak words of negativity and was always patient with each emailed question. She said, 'When you get pregnant' and not 'If you get pregnant.' It all was great from our first correspondence. It felt right and now we have a beautiful daughter in what seemed like such a simple and joyous journey.

"We are thankful and recommend Merciér Therapy to all women who are struggling."[2]

* * *

My philosophy, in a nutshell, is that when possible it's always worth it to first try gentler methods to conceive than to immediately turn to medicines that manipulate natural cycles by false and harsh means.

I do acknowledge and understand that medicine has helped many couples to conceive and deliver happy and healthy babies. However, my point is I would rather see a couple use more natural, gentler methods before the more extreme counterparts. In this book we'll delve into the world of Merciér Therapy, Reproductive Medicine, and the stories of the women I've worked with who've each endured a unique journey toward pregnancy.

My hope is that you'll find some peace within your own story by hearing the stories of others. Let's get started.

This book is written for the couples who long to take the least invasive approach possible. For the women who monitor their cycles and wait patiently to allow their bodies to do their job. There is much wisdom in nature, we as a culture are too quick to turn to unnatural, manipulative means. I feel this way even for and maybe especially if you've fallen into the sixtieth percentile of unexplained fertility challenges. And so you all know some of my personal story, I was in the fortieth percentile of these women with severe endometriosis and Hashimoto's thyroiditis. I chose to wait to see what my body was capable of before the rigamarole of the oft suggested harsh treatments. Besides, I also did not want the stress and pressure of the numerous scheduled tests and procedures. I chose not interference from the medical fertility realm, and I am so grateful that I trusted my own instincts.

In my years of practice, I have worked with quite a few couples who flatly refuse medical intervention. Some for religious reasons, others personal. And all of them had found the Merciér method to work inside their intentions. These couples would not even consider progesterone support in the luteal phase.[3] I have a great deal of respect for those who chose the path of least resistance. I believe in many cases, the body knows what to do, just sometimes it needs some help getting there. Nearly every single one of these couples who chose to conceive in the most natural way possible, through my methods, did go on to both become pregnant and deliver healthy babies.

For instance, in 2015 I had the pleasure of meeting Mike and Julie. They live in Wisconsin and decided to come to my practice in Illinois for the Shared Journey Fertility program.

Upon obtaining her gynecological history, I learned that Julie started her menses at age 13. Then at age 24 she started the Depo Provera contraceptive injection and stayed on for ten years. Julie decided to discontinue using the medication and after one year, her menses did not return. Irregular and/or excessive menstrual bleeding can diminish with long-term use of the contraceptive and it is common, or rather a high percentage of users become amenorrheic. The endometrium[4] becomes atrophic or "resting" with the prolongation of the therapy, and the period can cease altogether even.

Julie's gynecologist diagnosed her with iatrogenic amenorrhea and suggested using an oral contraceptive to encourage a period, but this did not work. She continued the use of the birth control pill for one year. Then after that year she did nothing and nothing happened. At this point Julie had been without her menses for sixteen years. I was astounded. This is the very first time that I have encountered a situation such as Julie's.

I learned that Julie underwent an hysterosalpingogram and both of her tubes were open. I also learned that her reproductive endocrinologist had set her on a plan of Menopur with an hCG trigger of ovulation and IUI (intrauterine insemination). Julie explained to me that she did not feel well while using Menopur and it felt as though she was "forcing her body to react."

Menopur (menotropins for injections) is a drug that contains follicle-stimulating hormone (FSH) that have been extracted from the urine of postmenopausal women. In short, these hormones are said to stimulate healthy ovaries to make eggs. The mechanism of action helps to grow a follicle that is optimal size for ovulation. During the injection process the egg grows to maturation inside of the follicle. At the same time a woman's estradiol levels are climbing to match the growth of the follicle and the endometrium is thickening with the rise of the estradiol.[5]

The first cycle did not produce a pregnancy, and though the couple wasn't thrilled about having another medically assisted cycle, they decided to try one more identical cycle. This time she became pregnant and delivered a healthy baby girl.

The couple did want to have another child, but this time they wanted to try something else. So they called me.

I did my magic on her reproductive organs and started her on a bio-identical hormone protocol. My goal was to gently encourage her to regain her menstrual cycle. I used a cycled approach of estriol and progesterone topical creams. Pretty soon, Julie started seeing her menses return, precisely the second month after starting the naturally prepared hormone regime. I was astounded. She was astounded. These hormones are gentle and produce such a nice result. No force inflicted and nothing that could pose potential unwanted side effects. I asked her to continue with cycling the creams and her menses continued.

Julie did continue using the bio-identical hormone regime, and close to three years after she received Merciér Therapy, Julie and Mike conceived. Julie's pregnancy was easy and uneventful. She had a healthy baby boy at age 43.[6]

There really is no need to panic that time is running short. I understand that for some their age is a major contributing factor or maybe they have a lesser egg reserve, but still, and I stress, panic will never be your friend.

I am here to help you fall in love with the process of allowing your body the space it needs to ebb and flow naturally. I always try to impress upon my patients that it is best to pump the brakes and allow God to make His provisions. Remember the little girl with the ladybugs? Rest your body, and expect a miracle. I do understand that for many this process is a bit more of a challenge because of life's complexities such as emotional trauma, physical trauma, relational or financial issues, or even something as simple as fine-tuning your diet to include more nutrients.

Utilizing the help of a Merciér trained professional will gently aid you in any scenario. We will liaise you through the rigors of emotional and physical problems while also teaching you how you can become proactive in the process. Ushering you to a conscious and gentle conception is our greatest goal. We strive to watch you grow as you honor and respect your body. We will tirelessly encourage you to give yourself what you need to support a pregnancy and to take the time to find the peace within the process.

This won't be another cheesy "how to" book. While I do consider myself an expert in the field of fertility, I am still humbled at the sheer number of women who in my twenty years of practice have trusted me with this most life-changing event, something as important and dear as growing their family. Teaching women how their body works and helping them make a clear decision is far more important to me than telling them what to do. It can be very challenging when trying to discern the best path for yourself and family but rest assured, we'll navigate these choppy waters together.

This is my calling. Time and time again it has been made abundantly clear that I am doing the work that God has intended for me. At least once a week I receive the happy news of a positive pregnancy through email, text, or phone call. Dozens of pictures of ovulation sticks, and I love every one of them. I know the long stories behind each of these positive pregnancy tests and what it took each woman to get to this point. At their core, I know these ladies have been pushing pianos up steep hills for so long in hopes of this moment, to feel the joy of this announcement. I am thrilled for all of them.

However, I know a whole new level of concern sets in as the pregnancy progresses and as the birth becomes imminent. The anxiety levels are still there until Mom's safely snuggling her healthy baby.

I am there through all of it. Every Merciér therapist is trained to be.

As a new mother there is an added feeling of accomplishment. She knows that she pursued the right path. The road has been a challenge to say the least. Running a marathon takes incredible dedication; the preparation alone is a full-time commitment and only a select few within that population have the drive to persevere because no one will run this race for you. You must endure the rigors of the training schedule, all the while minding your nutrition daily, on top of maintaining the strength and conditioning of your body physically, emotionally, and mentally to be your best. It's exhausting to even think about. My hat's off to all the ladies with the dedication and drive to make it happen. My patients inspire me every day.

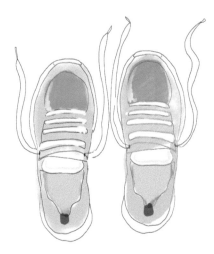

But let's try a thought experiment. Imagine signing up for the race and showing up the day of the race without the proper preparation. How do you think you would do? Terrible, probably. If I am talking about myself, there would be no way for me to run even a short distance. My lung capacity wouldn't be exercised and my metabolism wouldn't be calibrated to be able to handle smaller bits of food for fuel. My outlook would be one of a complete failure because I didn't show up for myself. I did not commit to the best possible outcome or even the most mediocre outcome.

IVF is a race that hopefully you will only have to endure once, so let's make sure that you're ready. As a Merciér therapist I will work deeply into your pelvis allowing your internal organs to move freely and receive fresh oxygenated blood to allow for optimal function. Does this make sense?

If you had an ankle injury would you ignore it and just go on training for the marathon hoping for the best? No way! You would not make it very far if you couldn't bear weight on one of your legs! Preparing your body for any rigorous activity is paramount, much like digging a solid foundation to build a house.

My work brings me great joy in knowing that women and men who consult with me say they feel like they are finally understood. I implement stress reduction techniques that will help bring them back to a place of control within their lives. A sense of control helps to eliminate the feelings of isolation that are common with infertility diagnoses.

While there are attractive and ever-evolving medical approaches to conceiving, they still do not always yield the desired outcome: a healthy baby. This process can be so painful both mentally and physically.

Typically, infertility patients struggle with negativity, lowered self-esteem, anger, insecurity, impatience, and fear. Life starts to become unrecognizable. The life of having a longed-for outcome becomes your every thought. Feelings of depression can start to set in. Some turn to medication, or worse. However, this is also an opportunity to help you understand and focus on your mental and physical experience.

Many times depression and anxiety are with you from long ago and stem from unresolved matters within your life before fertility even arose. But if you're on this journey, you and your partner really need each other right now. However, you both may be communicating with raw and defensive demeanors. Right when you should be getting along, you find you're at odds because you're so stressed. I want you to keep in mind that you are teammates and not enemies. We are biologically qualified to meet difficult challenges, even those that provoke disturbing internal conflict and confusion. Once you realize that you are struggling to become pregnant, you can regain a sense of self-control just by understanding how your body works.

Merciér Therapy empowers couples to recognize that they are not broken, and we're here to help you to take your power back. Working with a qualified professional who understands your struggle and will stay with you throughout your journey helps to create the support that you need. We will teach you how your body functions. For instance, like the signs of ovulation, what it means to have a shortened bleeding phase, an extensive surgical history, endometriosis, PCOS or a shortened cycle. We will dive deep into questions about your fertility history. Both yours and your husband's health, your habits that could be impeding a pregnancy. We will show you how you can effectively move forward in making positive changes within your life. We will teach you how to strengthen your own body to be more baby friendly.

Taking responsibility for your own fertility gives you agency. You'll feel stronger, clearer, more connected, more authentic, and more qualified to cope with whatever life is going to throw at you.

Even though all of this is your responsibility, I like to say that your ability to respond will become your response-ability.

Okay, let's make a baby!

And you begin again and sometimes you lose,
sometimes you win, but you begin again.
Even though your heart is breaking,
in time the sun will shine,
and you will begin again.

BARRY MANILOW

Chapter 1

MY JOURNEY

I learned about endometriosis in my early twenties. Back then I was a clinician at the Center for Human Reproduction in Chicago, and we treated many women with the disease. Endometriosis happens when the endometrium, the tissue that usually lines the inside of a woman's uterus, grows outside it. This tissue acts like regular uterine tissue does during your period: it will break apart and bleed at the end of the cycle. But this blood has nowhere to go. Surrounding areas may become inflamed or swollen. You might have scar tissue and lesions. It hurts like hell.

It appeared to me that the malady of endometriosis was both grim and aggressive, hopeless. Many women would attempt to become pregnant by using in vitro fertilization and often the results were not what they wanted. Once pregnant, pregnancy losses were seemingly more common. I noticed a significant issue concerning genetic issues that were incompatible with life and many more premature and preterm births.

I observed marital trouble, financial ruin, and emotional trauma. As an undergrad student learning the ways of Reproductive Endocrinology – as this is the medicine I wanted to eventually practice – I was learning how to perform semen analysis and intrauterine insemination, draw blood, and read pelvic ultrasound exams. It was an absolute privilege to monitor gonadotropin[7] and IVF cycles and to attend egg retrievals and embryo transfers. Spending time in the embryology lab with the embryologist fascinated me beyond words. I observed life in its most primitive form observing oocytes transform into fertilized eggs at the hand of a human and watching them then miraculously divide to make a glorious embryo. Taking the in-vivo process of conception outside of the body is pure awesome. The fact that we can even do such a thing says that we have come a long way in medicine.

However, in 1993 when I worked in the reproductive clinic IVF was only 19 years old. In my opinion there were many flaws.

In the United States in 1993 there were 31,718 IVF cycles for which the average charge was $6,233, leading to a total expenditure of approximately $197.70 million for IVF services in 1993.[8]

"Take-home baby" statistics reveals an even slimmer success rate than the advertised 15 percent. In 1991, of the women from whom eggs were retrieved, 15.2 percent went on to deliver a baby or babies (multiple births occur about 30 percent of the time). However, if you count women who started IVF cycles but did not yield eggs despite the drugs, the "success" rate drops to 12.5 percent per cycle; that is, only one in eight tries produced a baby. Turning the numbers around – something clinics generally avoid – yields this cold fact: in 1991, women endured 21,578 unsuccessful tries at IVF, or a failure rate of 87.5 percent.[9]

Nonetheless, the reproductive clinic was cranking out cycle after cycle and encouraging women who had failed their IVF cycle to keep trying more IVF. One cycle after another after another after another until there was no more insurance coverage, the funding ran out, or the cycle was too physically/mentally/emotionally arduous to continue. It wholly felt like a big business strictly seeking big revenue. I knew nothing different and figured other clinics operated the same way. Our clinic took new patients and they had come from one or more other reproductive endocrinology infertility clinics who described their past experiences as much the same as what we were offering. How many ways can medication and technology be used? Moreover, how are we going to send a woman with pelvic pain, explained or unexplained, through assisted reproductive technology? Shouldn't we be assessing the why first? What's the underlying cause of her fertility challenge? Is it her or could it be her partner? I can't tell you how many stories I've heard over my many years of practice where, after being examined by numerous reproductive endocrinologists, it had been discovered to be an issue with the male partner. It's a tragedy to undergo all that then find out it's too late for the woman to even think about building her family because at this point her eggs have aged beyond being able to fit the criteria for proceeding into an assisted cycle.

As an integrative doctor, I only refer to reproductive endocrinology practices that are very conscious of consulting with urology physicians to insure that all bases are covered thoroughly.

Around my time at the Center for Human Reproduction, I

was 22 and beginning to experience serious pelvic pain that was bad enough to send me to the emergency room on more than one occasion. I suffered from ruptured cysts, heavy bleeding, weight gain, fatigue, breast pain, headaches, pelvic and abdominal pain, gastrointestinal issues, and extreme abdominal bloating. These were my plagues that I felt through my menstruation and even throughout the rest of my cycle. It was unbearable.

There was a time I remember walking into Starbucks to get a cup of coffee. Prior to ordering I went to the ladies room just to empty my bladder, everything was fine, but when I walked out, quite suddenly, a wave of intense pelvic pain washed over me and I passed out from the sheer agony of it. I literally face planted onto the hard slate floor in front of a room full of strangers. I awoke to one of the employees asking me if I was okay. I was not okay and in fact could not move. EMS was called and off to the emergency room I went to discover that yet another cyst had ruptured. The feeling was so horrible that I felt it for days and days after. By urinating and relieving the fullness of my bladder it allowed for my uterus to move just enough that it disrupted the ovarian cyst from its position and voilà, that little movement from one organ to another caused a major problem.

As a young girl I would experience severe nose bleeds that would last full days. The blood that came out of my nose was not just red blood but resembled the menstrual blood that would later commence. I suffered half-dollar sized clots coming out of my nose as well as bright red fresh blood and the more mucus-tinged pink hues too, along with some other more worrisome fluids. My mother brought me in to the ENT twice to have my nose cauterized.

Later in my professional career I read a study stating that

endometrial tissue had been found in the brain and nasal cavities of cadavers. This really piqued my attention. Aggressive and hormonally sensitive tissue that grows with the ebb and flow of surging hormones can and will attach itself onto other very sensitive tissues such as gray matter, bowel, paranasal sinuses, and lung tissue. This could not be good.

Often the pain interfered with my daily routine. Both working and studying were becoming increasingly difficult. The symptoms were so wicked and debilitating that soon they took over my life. I, of course, turned to the profession that I was planning to enter: medicine. I visited with a well-respected OB/Gyn in which we often referred. My visit went well, I remember being hopeful. Pelvic exam and PAP smear was normal, and I was prescribed an oral contraceptive. I took the pill for three or so cycles when it became clear that they were causing severe hormonal headaches. The headaches were so intense that I wanted to die, and I looked to medicine again to help me. The answer was to stay on the pill and add an injectable drug (Sumatriptan) to help combat the pain of these headaches. I used the medication, and it helped, but ironically the side effect of the headache medicine is a headache. It was at this time that I started thinking about my future in allopathic medicine and found an educational program at the Chicago School of Massage Therapy. I slowly but surely tapered my schedule to a minimum at the fertility clinic and enrolled into a professional massage therapy certificate program. It was there that I learned a wealth of knowledge about anatomy and physiology of the human body. This was exactly the place I needed to be studying. I loved it so much. At the time of completion from my undergrad program and massage school, I had applied to the Spartan Health Sciences University

Medical School in St. Lucia and was accepted. But in my mind and heart I felt a strong calling to a path of natural healing modalities.

I decided to listen to my instincts and explore my options, and while doing so I decided to take a class entitled Bodywork for the Childbearing Year. In this class we learned how to apply therapeutic massage for the pre and post natal periods. At some point in the class the instructor, Kate Jordan, began talking about doulas and midwives, here is where my heart flew alight. I was thoroughly intrigued and felt an undeniable pull towards the service of women as a doula.

Soon after, I joined the organization Doulas of North America. I worked directly with nurse midwives, Glenda Embry and Karen Wexler at Sherman Hospital in Elgin, Illinois. There, I would offer my doula services to the mothers who were alone during their labor and birth, nearly all of them were eager for the help. I was young, had not yet gone through a pregnancy myself, but with each labor and delivery, I knew this was where I wanted to be. Watching women transition into motherhood still moves me to this day. The tensions and the anticipation of giving birth alone were palpable. I felt that this was my place.

My doula work quickly led me into midwifery training. My first taste of possibly becoming a midwife was in 1998 when I stayed at the home of a Shari Daniels, CPM in Miami, Florida. Shari owned the birth center next to her home. Many babies were born each month at the Miami Beach Maternity Center. It was an exciting job. Our phone would ring all hours of the night and we would have to rush next door to the birth center whenever duty called. Watching a seasoned midwife attend a woman in labor and be able to reassure her that all was well with her and her baby and witnessing the miracle of birth moved me beyond words. I was in love with my choice and the practice. I had made the right decision.

The training path wasn't the easiest – long hours, difficult and unexpected scenarios, and not to mention the grand amount of responsibility of managing the life of a mother and her unborn baby – but with great tribulations comes great reward.

From Miami my training then continued to Kingston, Jamaica. There, I studied with author and revolutionary midwife, Nancy Wainer, CPM, known for coining the term VBAC (Vaginal Birth After Cesarean) but also co-cofounded the first cesarean prevention organization in the world and was instrumental in the formation of the Cesarean Prevention Movement. I had the opportunity to work with Nancy in 1998 as a student midwife in the Victoria Jubilee hospital. We served women in labor, during their birth, and in the postnatal period. The Jamaican women were strong and robust, just really amazing at birthing babies. I felt privileged to serve them in their hospital.

Next stop was Summertown, Tennessee where I studied Advanced Midwifery skills with The Farm Midwives. Yes, I worked with Ina May Gaskin, Pamela Hunt, Joanne Santana, Deborah Flowers and Carol Nelson. It was a great honor and privilege to have listened to these women's wisdom as they shared their amazing knowledge of midwifery. I have a picture of me with Ina May showing me how to maneuver a breech baby if I would ever need that skill. What an awesome delight!

Finally, my studies then continued and concluded at Casa De Nacimiento in El Paso, Texas where I ultimately finished my training and then practiced as a home birth midwife for 12 years. While practicing midwifery I decided to attend a small dual Naturopathic/

PhD program at Central States College of Health Sciences. There, I took classes to further my studies in natural medicine concurrently while practicing as a home birth midwife. At this time, my endometriosis still raged on. I started using my own self-made deep visceral manipulation sequence for nagging pelvic pain, which gave me a great deal of relief, but the pain kept returning. I felt that I was onto something but was just not able to work deeply enough on myself to fully alleviate my symptoms. It became plain that I needed someone else to assist me. It was now 2005 and the Merciér Therapy thought process had begun.

I graduated from my dual ND/PhD program in 2007 and began to think again seriously about a career in fertility. While reading the current stats back in 2006, it appeared to me that nothing significant had changed in the medical model of fertility treatment.[10]

By this time, I'd already had two pelvic surgeries and still suffered a tremendous amount of pelvic pain. I knew that I wanted to pursue motherhood in my future but was scared that I might fall under the tragic statistic of women who seem infertile due to the disease. Well, time progressed, and my pelvic pain was escalating out of control. An ultrasound revealed an endometrioma on my left ovary again and it was slowly leaking fluid into my pelvic cavity behind my uterus. I endured a third laparoscopy to have the mass removed and by that time I was married. My then-husband and I were told post-operative that my organs were in terrible shape and that I'd need to have in vitro fertilization if we wanted to have a baby. My reply to the surgeon was that I was not going to do IVF, but rather try some different things first. I knew the inner workings of IVF and felt that it was not for me. But more so, I thought I could pursue my research into gentle yet deep pelvic visceral manipulation.

At this time, concurrently with my practice, I was an instructor at Everest College teaching anatomy and physiology. Our organs are so neatly compact and organized in the body, merely contacting the pelvic organs seemed like such an obvious solution, quite frankly I was shocked it hadn't been tried before.

I had a group of my students work on me using the Merciér Therapy methods and my husband and I had conceived the next cycle without intervention! Each and every time I say that story a shiver goes up my spine.

Remember, I was told that I wouldn't get pregnant without the use of IVF. You can imagine how it felt to call the surgeon who did my third laparoscopy and let him know that I was pregnant! It was awesome going in to his office for an early ultrasound to see that sweet little heartbeat, and while I was overjoyed and preoccupied with my little one, my own heart couldn't help but do a little jig that my method worked, that I had beaten the odds and shown there was another way, a natural way. That IVF is not always the answer.

Have you ever placed a headband in your hair and just an hour later felt a slight tension in the back of your head? How about after a shower and you feel that a hair might be tied around your toe? These examples may sound silly but your body is very sensitive. Now imagine that we dial up the amperage on your endocrine system repeatedly. One might think that because the medications given during a medically assisted cycle are prescribed that they are safe. Yes, your cycles will be monitored to ensure that you are not floating into the danger zone. Yes, they are prescribed by a medical doctor and are generally deemed as safe. However, using drugs to stimulate your endocrine system can create a scenario in which your body does not recover. This is especially true if there are already issues such as diabetes, thyroid issues, Addison's disease, and Cushing's syndrome. The change in your health status could be minute and unnoticeable, or something bigger could be lurking and starting to wreak havoc silently. Sometimes patients find that something very blatant has changed but they cannot pinpoint the source and they continue the medication, unknowing that it's actually making them sick.

Any time we put a substance in to our body there is bound to be a biological change that occurs. For instance, using an antibiotic will change the environment of the microbiome, which can cause long term health implications such as inflammatory bowel disease, or can even reduce the ability of immune cells to kill bacteria, and changes to the biochemical environment directly elicited by treatment can protect the bacterial pathogen. Oy.

Sadly, I lost that pregnancy at 8 weeks, but I did get pregnant again within four months of that loss. We had a heartbeat for that pregnancy as well and lost that one too at 10 weeks. Because of all the surgery and trauma that I'd already experienced, I decided on expectant management for both losses. In other words, I chose to wait for my body to miscarry naturally. The first loss happened on its own very gently without a lot of blood loss or pain. The second loss was not as easy. I waited for two weeks for the miscarriage to start and there was a great deal of blood loss. It became clear that I did need a D&C.[11] Talk about heartbreak. Ultimately, it is best to wait for your body to pass the pregnancy naturally. Many medical providers will urge you to schedule a D&C quickly to remove the tissue. However, a D&C is surgery and can cause scar tissue on the inside of the uterus. There is also a 20% risk of Asherman's syndrome post D&C that can cause adhesions to form inside of the uterus.

Asherman's is considered rare because it often goes undiagnosed. Ultimately, scar tissue can inhibit a pregnancy from implanting, meaning someone already suffering from infertility challenges may not want to add any negative impact to her chances.

My third pregnancy was the charm and come fall my first-born baby was due. I planned on a home birth. My midwife friend and colleague, Hillary Keiser, CNM cared for me and instilled lots of tender loving care. My prenatal care was wonderful. I felt loved and cared for, which is paramount for a relaxed and success-ful home birth.

At this time I was 37 and my pregnancy was uneventful, but at my 39 week and 4 day appointment my baby was determined to be breech. I went in for an ultrasound to confirm the baby's position and her head was under the right side of my ribcage. Confirmed breech. I crawled on my hands and knees trying to encourage her to move but by this time she was too big to move. My obstetrician, Kevin Hussey, MD and I talked about doing an external version but even with this procedure he was not convinced that she'd turn and being that she was so wedged up there, he concluded it was too risky and we risked tearing the placenta. It was not worth trying in my opinion. My midwife and mommy intuition played a huge role here. I worked so hard for this baby and was not willing to put her in any undue stress. Usually, a baby can be born breech if a mother has had one or more vaginal births prior, she could try to push a breech baby through the pelvis. The pathway has been paved before and thus it is easier for the baby's body to come through without as much issue. But this is not always the case.

In the end, my brilliant Clair Celine was born safely via c-section on October 20, 2011.

When Clair was 18 months old, I could feel in my heart that I wanted to have another baby. Initially, both my husband and I felt that one child was going to be best for our family, but I changed my mind. We embarked upon trying for baby number two and ended up losing three more pregnancies, all with heartbeats. My estradiol could not climb high enough to support the growing embryo and then it would peter out and I'd lose the pregnancy. Estradiol forms the vital organs (heart and spinal cord) of the baby. Also, because I had had a c-section I was suffering from secondary fertility challenges possibly due to organ immobility as well.

But thank the Lord, my seventh pregnancy turned out to be healthy and strong.

Ultimately, I sought out the help of my friend Zvi Binor, MD, a reproductive endocrinologist, and let him know that I needed his help in keeping my next baby. We decided on using an injectable follicle stimulating hormone, ultrasound/blood monitoring, hCG trigger, and a timed intercourse cycle. Due to the last pregnancy loss, and prior to starting any treatment, I'd need to have a sono-hysterogram (saline ultrasound) to ensure that my uterine cavity was empty and ready to receive a pregnancy.[12] All the while each day my husband would deeply manipulate my uterus each night prior to starting the injections. I could feel that the endometriosis was starting to ease-up and soon I could feel the movements of my uterus much easier. This time, I felt well prepared for my gentle medically assisted cycle.

I was cleared to start my cycle and as a result I grew a beautiful follicle which resulted in a healthy pregnancy. As the end of my pregnancy grew nearer I really had held in my mind to try to birth vaginally. As a midwife I had attended many HBACs (Home Birth After Cesarean section) and observed that these women did very well and had a lovely deep sense of accomplishment too. And now, many physicians are encouraging VBACs.

At this time, I was 40 and very healthy. I grew a healthy baby and was set on a VBAC. At 38 weeks my water broke on its own and labor commenced. I labored for sixteen hours and my baby stayed high in my pelvis at a negative two station *and* I only dilated to four. I felt that after all that time without change my baby was sending me a message that I interpreted as a sign of needing to be born. My sweet son, Seth, was born via c-section on June 3rd, 2014 and had a tight and short double cord around his neck. It's no wonder he was hung up too high and never descended. Nonetheless, I just endured another pelvic surgery.

A description of my healing would be fair overall. After my surgical birth with Clair I developed a seroma[13] at the incision directly right of the pubic symphysis. However, I consider myself to be very sensitive and I ended up going back to the hospital to have an interventional radiologist drain the fluid and place a drain into the pouch so the fluid would not collect again. The drain was removed one week after it was placed and the outcome uneventful.

As the months went on during the post partum period I could feel that my pelvis was completely immobile and in fact felt very "stuck". My menses actually returned when I was 6 weeks post partum with my daughter, and now same with my son. While prior to my first pregnancy I experienced a deep visceral cyclic pelvic pain, it was not present post either c-section. I firmly believe that this was due to my intense work and preparation prior to both healthy pregnancies.

I am so grateful for my two wonderful children. I am grateful for my midwives, doctors, students, my first fellow Merciér Therapists.

Nature gives to every time and season some beauties of its own; and from morning to night, as from the cradle to the grave, it is but a succession of changes so gentle and easy that we can scarcely mark their progress.

CHARLES DICKENS

Chapter 2

THE MERCIÉR THERAPY METHOD

Whether you're suffering from a fertility challenge, pelvic pain or a past trauma, I will help you to navigate your way to making a choice to help yourself and start to heal. Movement equals life. This I know to be true.

Merciér Therapy is a site specific, deep pelvic organ manipulation that encourages blood flow and organ movement.

When we do this manual work, we encourage optimal pelvic organ wellness.

Organs need to be fully mobile to do their job. Things like scar tissue can glue organs in place disallowing movement. And less movement equals less blood flow.

As part of the treatment, I give my patients a journal in

which to record their cycles so we can recognize consistencies and inconsistencies. It's a good idea to put pen to paper and write down what's going on. This not only ignites your right brain, the creative side, but helps me see patterns.

For several years prior to creating my new modality and giving it a name, I thought about the pelvic organs in relation to the ebb and flow of movement throughout a woman's hormone cycle. The uterus lifts high into the pelvis during ovulation to enable the uterine tubes (fallopian tubes) to align in accordance with the impending follicular rupture (ovulation). Once ovulation occurs, the end of the uterine tube (fimbria) must contract in peristalsis to receive the egg. Poetically, the tube waves the egg inward in a flowy sort of motion.

Now remember, when there is poor organ mobility there is poor overall organ function and blood flow. Any organ or body part that is restricted in movement is probably not functioning optimally. Surgical scar tissue can lock organs into a fixed position causing moderate to severe restriction and disallowing for optimal overall function. When constructing Merciér Therapy's methods, I kept in mind the analogy that if we were to undergo any type of orthopaedic or cardiac surgery then we'd need physical rehabilitation to return to a pre-operative status. The same is such with the pelvic organs post-operative with the same therapeutic end goal in mind.

When consulting with a woman at age 35 or beyond, I give a very simple scenario that is very easy to understand: think about having a house guest. It is morning and your houseguest is upstairs and still asleep. You're starting to make breakfast downstairs and the first thing you do is cook the bacon.

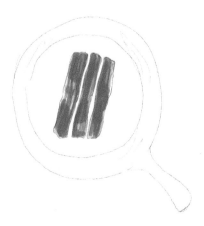

Bacon is not only a strong, greasy scent but a familiar one that we associate with breakfast. As the bacon cooks, the aroma starts to make its way up to your houseguest. She smells it and it smells yummy but she still isn't ready to wake up just yet. Next you start a pot of coffee, another universal scent associated with breakfast. But your guest remains sleepy. You go to the bottom of the stairs and announce, "Breakfast is ready!" But alas, nothing.

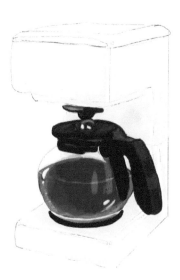

Finally, you go upstairs and gently say: "Good morning, breakfast is ready." And still, she doesn't even try to wake. Gently, you lay your hand on your sleepy guest and give a little shake. "Breakfast is ready."

That gentle nudge is most times enough for sleepyhead to awaken. I liken this example to what Merciér Therapy will do. By gently contacting and manipulating the ovarian surface, the movement essentially wakes the area up so that your ovaries are able to hear the finely orchestrated dance of the endocrine system, thus alerting them that it's time to make estradiol.

In post-therapy session mid-cycle estradiol levels, I have seen marked improvements. My theory is that the work done on the ovaries has turned on the light switch, so now everything functions and dances in communication once again.

Another example: say you have your gall bladder removed. The surgeon lifts your liver to be able to access the gall bladder, and once removed, the liver is carefully returned to its position and you are closed back up. Will there be scar tissue forming? Yes. Are you sent to do any therapy to help you recover? No. How about this? You give birth via c-section, just as I did with both of my babies, and your bladder is retracted away from your uterus so that the incision can be made to remove your baby. Once the baby and placenta are removed, your uterus is taken outside of your body and placed on your abdomen to be repaired then neatly replaced back inside of your pelvis and your abdomen is closed. Voilà! Your pelvic organs should function normally for the rest of your days without one bit of rehabilitation. Nope. This is not how it works, my friends. It is 100% true that women are not being steered toward a path of ultimate healing.

Now, let's talk more about the surgical birth.

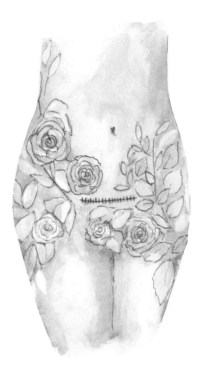

Cesarean section is a lifesaving discovery. Many women have lost their lives back in the day when this kind of surgery was impossible. However, people forget that even though it's common, it's still a major surgery, and one quite often over-used. It should only be used in the event that it becomes necessary, but even so, it leaves serious scar tissue in its wake. Remembering what we discussed earlier, you can imagine how the entire pelvis and abdominal region is affected. The lower anterior uterine wall is incised to remove the baby and once repaired it is placed back into the pelvis where it hugs the bladder. Scar tissue can form between the two organs making both immobile thus decreasing blood flow to both. I've spoken to women who – even after a quarter of a century – post c-section have had to undergo additional surgery to remove scar tissue that had attached itself to the pelvic organs and surrounding structures causing severe organ pain and dysfunction. I believe that when scar tissue is left untreated it can cause longer term damage to both the surgically incised organs and the area around the incisions such as the muscles, ligaments, and fascia.

I am more than familiar with gynecologic surgery as I've had three laparoscopies, two D&Cs, and two c-sections. Women that have undergone at least one surgical procedure have the risk of scar tissue being present. Scar tissue is the body's way of healing and protecting; however, it can, over time, cause damage if not addressed within a 5-month time period post-operative. Once that 5-month window has passed, the body starts to accept the new "normal" positioning. Can the body function? Yes. Can the body function as efficiently and optimally as prior to the surgery? No. You may wonder, that if the body were functioning at its optimum prior to surgery, then why would it not adapt to the "new" normal and make provisions to accept that change? Okay. If surgery is indicated, then typically there is a presence that needs examining and indeed the body was not at all functioning at its best. Merciér Therapy gets into that space and helps it adapt better after the trauma.

Blood flow is the essence of healing and healthy tissue, and that's essentially the heart of our work, making the blood flow, getting everything back to normal.

To encourage movement within the pelvis, we must apply a visceral manipulative protocol to work deeply. We want to release the tensions created by scar tissue because if left untreated it will be forcing structures into odd and ineffective positions. Breaking through the scar tissue, and getting blood to return to the area will help your reproductive system function at its most effective. When performed correctly, Merciér Therapy and your body work together to perform nothing short of synergetic magic.

Medicine and integrative practice both have their place, but for me, I will always stress natural methods first. If your sink needs a new washer, you do not go out and remodel the whole bathroom without seeing if a simple fix would do the trick.

At this time, it is worth noting too, that I personally train all of my Merciér Therapists. I love my practice and I love serving my patients as much as Mercier Therapists do theirs. Collaboration is the only way I can service all the women of the world who need this therapy. It has been a wonderful honor and privilege to see Merciér Therapy applied all over the world from the Netherlands to the Middle East. The Mercier tribe has been accepted by the medical community so long as I draw clear distinction between what I do and what they do. I never want to drive a wedge between us and negate medicine for what it contributes to women experiencing pelvic pain or fertility challenges. However, what I do want to do is be helpful in creating solid solutions for physicians to refer their patients and know that Merciér Therapy is valid as a therapy.

My experience in working with medical professionals has been good. They are always intrigued with how manipulation can help repair and maintain proper organ function. In fact, I have traveled around the world presenting my research at varying professional conferences, and while in Dubai, I was approached by an anatomy professor from the University of New England College of Osteopathic Medicine. He said that he read my abstract and asked me to tell him more about my work. I explained my theory on improving organ movement and thus enhancing overall organ function and blood flow. He looked at me like my hair was on fire and said, "That is absolutely brilliant!" I will anecdotally add that I was 7 weeks pregnant with my son while in the U.A.E. and I was very nauseated. The only thing I could eat while there was yogurt and fruit. So here I am talking with this PhD level anatomist whilst having a lovely lunch served to us and all I wanted to do is vomit! It was horrible, but I was so honored that this awesome professor agreed 100% with my explanation on organ function optimization.

I can recall a gynecologist who once referred her toughest case to me. The woman was 56, an attorney who worked long hours, never had any children, and complained of urinary incontinence for years. The referring physician explained to me that her patient suffered from a grade 2 cystocele. A cystocele is a prolapse of the bladder against the anterior vaginal wall. The issue became so intolerable that the doctor suggested performing a bladder sling and the patient decided against it. I was her last resort prior to undergoing surgery. Bless you, sweet gynecologist, for offering the best solution within your tool bag.

Upon my first visit with Susan[14], I noticed that her core muscles were very weak. I asked her if she did any kind of strength training exercises and she said that she took long walks each weekend and that was all that she had time to do. I did an external pelvic organ mobility evaluation to find that her uterus was in a fixed anteflexed position, which was also confirmed by ultrasound. Anteflexion means that the uterus flips forward exaggeratedly toward the pubis, hugging the bladder tightly and most times does not allow the bladder to fill to a normal volume. A little bit of urine can irritate the incredibly shrinking bladder space and the weakness of the core can contribute to a prolapse. I started my work to pull the uterus out of its fixed and restricted position to incorporate more organ movement and help to restore blood flow. At the end of each treatment, I used a therapeutic tape to create a sling-like structure on her lower pelvis and abdomen in order to provide support. We did this same treatment for one hour each week for six weeks. We also searched for a pilates studio that was close to her home so she could commit to core training as self-preservation. After a spell, I noticed marked overall improvement of the organ mobility as well as Susan's experience of not needing to wear heavy protection during her day any longer. She could finally be free of feeling embarrassment, her confidence was restored. I am happy to say that she did not opt for surgery and instead did what I asked of her with core strength training. If that had not worked, my other option was to ask her gynecologist about getting fitted for a pessary[15], but thankfully, it didn't have to come to that either.

Sometimes women will come to see me and ask if it is my opinion to continue with other holistic practitioners along with working with me. If we can all work well and in concert, then of course, yes, but if we are causing stress due to multiple visits and time spent then it's not necessary as Merciér Therapy is an all-encompassing holistic practice. Together, we will find your hormonal imbalances, along with any nutritional deficiencies as well. But I will be honest, I have little knowledge of Chinese medicines and herbs and would not feel comfortable saying yes to them alongside my work, considering we'll be working with our own supplements and (possibly) hormones. Releasing as much stress as possible is the best, but always talk with your doctor and practitioners if you have any concerns.

We live in a society exquisitely dependent on science and technology, in which hardly anyone knows anything about science and technology.

CARL SAGAN

Chapter 3

SCIENCE OF THE PRACTICE

A pregnancy in harmony is a pregnancy that was probably carefully planned for in advance. For instance, barreling through pelvic pain into a pregnancy sometimes cannot be avoided and just naturally happens. However, if there is an issue of pelvic discomfort or disharmony from a hormonal or physical perspective then these issues must be addressed prior to conceiving. By eliminating an issue that could potentially cause trouble you are all the wiser to prepare.

Many couples seek out consultation with me after they've failed multiple rounds of medical interventions. When these interventions fail, women can be left feeling defeated and broken.

I wish that these women had found me prior to squandering

precious time, emotions, and resources, because here is the thing, dear sister, *you're not broken.* There is a glitch in the system somewhere. Take the extra time to figure out the glitch otherwise you will be living by the definition of insanity.

A woman is born with all the eggs she will ever have, which at birth is typically around one million. By puberty, she usually has half that – and each month after puberty, she loses up to one thousand eggs. Of those, only one egg is matured and ovulated each month. With age, egg quality is diminished over time, as a woman is exposed to all the inevitable forces of everyday life – illness, toxins, free-radicals, fever, and more – that can damage the DNA inside her eggs. That's why, as a woman gets older, it's more likely that she'll have genetically abnormal eggs, which can decrease the chances of a viable fertilization, and increase the chances of both miscarriage and genetic disorders for the baby.

For the women who do achieve pregnancy, the chance of genetic abnormality – resulting in miscarriage or chromosomal disorders like Down Syndrome – increases exponentially as a woman ages.[16] This is why women choose to freeze their eggs in their twenties or early thirties, because those eggs are much more likely to result in a healthy pregnancy, even when used later.

I like to use the simple example of how many eggs you have left by age in the following graphics. These are just examples and do not represent every woman who seeks to become pregnant.

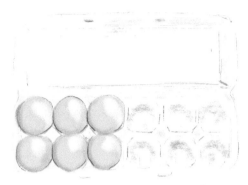

Example of how many eggs you may have at age 35. Ovulating a quality egg every other cycle which is why it seems like it may take longer to conceive.

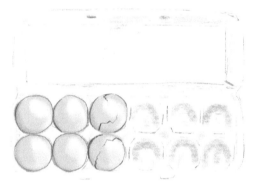

Example of a woman approaching her 40th year and maybe there are only 4 good quality eggs to ovulate and 2 poorer quality eggs that may ovulate and fertilitze yet could result in miscarriage.

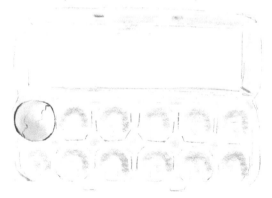

Example of a woman's reserve after age 42. There are a few eggs left but they may be of very poor quality therefore resulting in genetic abnormalities and potentially more miscarriages.

Let's take a look at a few tests to determine potential egg quality and overall reserve:

The first test, the Anti-Müllerian Hormone test or AMH, the protein hormone produced by special cells inside the ovarian follicles. The level of AMH in the blood can help doctors estimate the number of follicles inside the ovaries, and, therefore, the woman's egg count. A typical AMH level for a fertile woman is 1.0–4.0 ng/ml; under 1.0 ng/ml is considered low and indicative of a diminished ovarian reserve.[17]

The other test we use is Follicle Stimulating Hormone. FSH is tested between days 2-4 of your menstrual cycle to gain an idea of what might be happening with your reserve. When your FSH levels are abnormally high, this is because the eggs in your ovaries are not maturing at normal levels of FSH. Your body tries to fix the problem by increasing FSH until (hopefully) the eggs mature. With IVF or injectable fertility drugs, the hormone FSH is being injected to stimulate your ovaries. But just like your ovaries aren't responding to your natural FSH, they also are unlikely to respond to injected FSH. Injected FSH is used with both non IVF and IVF cycles.

FSH works on a feedback loop with estrogen. As FSH tells the eggs in your ovaries to grow, the eggs release estrogen in response. As the follicles (or eggs) get bigger, they release more estrogen. The higher levels of estrogen stimulate your reproductive system to slow down the release of FSH. In other words, FSH levels will naturally drop as the follicles get bigger and eggs in the ovary mature. If the eggs don't start to mature and release estrogen, then FSH levels won't drop. In fact, your body will release higher and higher levels of FSH in a desperate attempt to stimulate egg development.

In a woman with good ovarian reserves, properly dosed FSH

injected hormone will lead to strong egg growth in her ovaries. In a woman with poor ovarian reserves, the ovaries will not respond as well and higher dosed FSH becomes necessary.

Women with very low AMH and high FSH levels have not done well with an IVF cycle and probably should not undergo such a cycle due to poor outcomes and possible cycle cancellation. Many women in this scenario are typically guided toward using donor eggs and then have better outcomes.

The difference in egg quality between a 25-year-old and a 40-year-old is a matter of the statistical likelihood of the one egg she's ovulated being normal. Because women in their late 30s and 40s have a higher percentage of abnormal eggs, it's much more likely that their one egg each month will be abnormal. That's why natural fertility declines with age, and why we see infertility, miscarriage, and genetic disorders more often with women over 35.

In some cases young women have what's called premature ovarian aging, a condition in which ovaries stop functioning prematurely, leading to a low number of good-quality eggs. This is where DHEA can make a difference.

Let's make this simple. You'll start off in your twenties with a full egg carton which represents nicely twelve eggs for twelve ovulation cycles in one year. Beginning in our thirties, the rate of egg production falls, and women will lose quite a lot of good quality eggs, soon being left with possibly as few as six good eggs per year. Late in our thirties and early forties we will have a steep decline in reserves, yielding only some good eggs and a few poorer in quality. The poorer quality eggs may fertilize but the chance of survival is small or may bear a genetic disorder. Around our early forties there is still the chance of ovulating healthy eggs but this is almost completely dependent on the women's health. However, and in most cases, there is such a small reserve that we've got to improve blood flow and organ movement to help ensure that the remaining eggs have the opportunity to be utilized. Higher-quality embryos are less likely to be miscarried.

So what do you do with a dwindling reserve and numbers that suggest that your eggs are on the decline? I typically use the DHEA protocol with some bio-identical hormone supplementation and a Merciér twist.

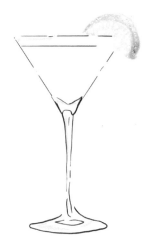

DEHYDROEPIANDROSTERONE (DHEA)

DHEA is a natural sex hormone produced in the human body. It is used as a precursor to other sex hormones such as estrogen and testosterone which are needed for reproduction. DHEA production peaks in a woman's twenties and naturally declines as she gets older.

The research to date on DHEA's egg health effects has been impressive, showing it can help improve diminished ovarian reserve.

Research also shows a strong connection between DHEA and fertility. Current thinking is that DHEA may actually help women conceive. This is really encouraging, especially in light of it being both safe and natural.

Among women taking DHEA, fertility may improve due to an increase in the number of "good-quality" eggs available for fertilization. In an independent study, Israeli researchers recruited 33 women who had difficulty conceiving. They were randomly split into two groups, one control and one treatment, with the treatment group receiving 75 mg of DHEA daily. All women eventually underwent IVF (in vitro fertilization) treatments.[18]

Supplementation began at least six weeks before IVF and continued for up to five months. The result: women taking DHEA were three times more likely to conceive. In addition, there was a 23% live birth rate in the treatment group compared to a 4% rate in the control group.

The mechanism of action is not entirely known, but it is believed that DHEA increases overall ovarian response during a cycle. Hence increasing the number of good-quality eggs. So, women who are actively trying to conceive may want to keep this in mind, especially women in their late thirties and early forties.

Additional studies also show the benefits of taking DHEA for fertility, with one recent study demonstrating improved ovarian function in women over forty.[19]

If my patient has poor egg quality, diminished reserve, or ovarian failure then I generally suggest using the DHEA at 75mg per day along with Pregnenolone 30mg per day during the conception period. Using the two hormones together will form a synergy to help create a stronger benefit for the women who use them. Though I don't like to use this combo beyond a six-month timeframe and will reevaluate at that point. DHEA can be used for prolonged periods along with Pregnenolone in lower doses.

Also, Pregnenolone counteracts the potential masculinizing effects of DHEA. In this regard, it may be more important than DHEA for a woman's hormonal balance. Long-time DHEA researcher, William Regelson, writes that some researchers who have pondered the question of whether Pregnenolone alone is able to reverse the age-related decline of all "superhormones" (including progesterone and estrogen) believe that "a combination of Pregnenolone and DHEA working together will do the trick."[20] In other words, these two hormones appear to work in harmony. Given the upside and support from a growing body of literature, it makes good sense to take them along with progesterone during the luteal phase.

* * *

DHEA is a naturally existing hormone that the female body converts into androgens, mainly testosterone. Even though androgens are male hormones, they're present in both sexes and are essential in the female body for the production and development of healthy eggs. DHEA is used primarily to treat women with diminished ovarian reserve which occurs either because of premature ovarian failure or female aging.

DHEA's beneficial effects on female fertility include:

- Increased IVF pregnancy rates

- Increased chance of spontaneous conceptions

- Shortened time to pregnancy

- Increased quality and quantity of eggs and embryos

- Decreased risk of miscarriage and decreased chromosomal abnormalities in embryos

- Improved cumulative pregnancy rates in patients under fertility treatment

While it is important to focus on egg health, DHEA may not be the correct choice for you. For instance, if you have polycystic ovary syndrome (PCOS) and your androgens are elevated already, then this would not be appropriate for you. DHEA will further that excess burden and could potentially cause your disease to progress and your symptoms to become much worse.

Ultimately, I urge you to please work with a provider who is familiar with the DHEA protocol. I use it in my practice but not unopposed with a few other goodies to support its function and utilization.

PROGESTERONE

Progesterone is a miracle hormone. It is in abundance in a woman's body post ovulation. After ovulation, the hormone spikes to keep the uterus relaxed so the pregnancy can implant. It can be taken synthetically to increase the likelihood of pregnancy; however, used incorrectly during the cycle, it can inhibit ovulation.

Progesterone can come in several forms. I always first recommend a naturally derived product to be applied topically. When used via transdermal application, the hormone is picked up and taken directly into the bloodstream, as opposed to the oral route, where it is going through the liver and then coated with a protein. In other words, the oral route may not give you the dose that you need. During an IVF or FET cycle, the physician may choose to use a few different applications for delivering the hormone. Oral is one, vaginal is another, and, finally, injectable is most popular with IVF. Many times there are a few combinations with regard to medically assisted cycles.

Just a step further to explain what a micronized hormone means and why it may be a better choice. Typically, medicine uses the type of progesterone that is synthesized into tiny particles and suspended in an oil to be delivered into the small intestine where it will be absorbed and readily available for use. Prometrium is a prescription and is by far my favorite and can be used orally and vaginally. I love this so much!

Progesterone is the hormone that helps block the detrimental effects of estrogen, such as menstrual cramps, breast tenderness, and PMS in those women who are menstruating, along with fibroids, endometriosis, PCOS, and fibrocystic disease of the breast. It is also known to help eliminate asthma symptoms, lessen migraine headache episodes, and decrease morning sickness. In addition, it helps to prevent all cancers caused by estrogen, such as cancers of the breast, uterus, ovaries, cervix, colon, and the prostate in men.

Progesterone also has a profound effect on insulin. Insulin is a hormone that is associated with the causation of obesity as well as type II diabetes and its many complications. It is a fact that insulin raises blood pressure and is felt to be a major influence in speeding up the aging process. Progesterone blocks insulin receptor sites on cells, thereby helping to eliminate drops in blood sugar (hypoglycemia). As a result, it prevents sleepiness after eating, between 3 and 4 PM, and while driving. This ability to block the effects of insulin also helps with weight loss.

Lastly, progesterone blocks the action and over-production of adrenaline. Adrenaline is popularly known as the "fight-or-flight" hormone, and excess levels can create anger, road rage, insomnia, restless leg syndrome, and teeth grinding. When anger is internalized, it can lead to depression, anxiety, fibromyalgia, irritable bowel syndrome (IBS), plus other problems. As a neurotransmitter in the brain, adrenaline can cause the mind to race, which can cause problems with focusing – i.e. attention deficit hyperactivity disorder (ADHD) or "brain fog." Adrenaline also causes urinary urgency in adults as well as bed-wetting in children. Leg cramps at night are also caused by adrenaline, and can usually be relieved within 30-60 seconds when progesterone is applied to the area of cramping.

For what it's worth, I would bet that adrenaline is probably the number one cause of unexplained weight gain. Increased stress stimulates our adrenal glands to produce excessive and inadequate amounts of these hormones, causing some to overeat, stress eat, and others to abstain. Levels of the "stress hormone," cortisol, rise during tension-filled times. This can turn your overeating into a habit. Because increased levels of the hormone also help cause higher insulin levels, your blood sugar drops and you crave sugary, fatty foods.

CLOMIPHENE CITRATE (CLOMID)

Clomiphene citrate, more commonly known by its brand names Clomid and Serophene, is a medication prescribed to women to stimulate ovulation in order to treat infertility. It stimulates ovulation in women who do not ovulate or ovulate irregularly. This drug was created by Frank Palopoli in 1956 while he worked for Merrell Company. It first successfully induced ovulation in women in 1961 and was approved by the Food and Drug Administration (FDA) in 1967. This medication can be used to help women conceive naturally, to time ovulation for intrauterine insemination, or to stimulate the maturation of eggs to be extracted and used in procedures such as in vitro fertilization (IVF), gamete intrafallopian transfer (GIFT), and zygote intrafallopian transfer (ZIFT).

Women with higher than normal levels of male hormones, known as hyperandrogenism, are good candidates for clomiphene therapy as are women with normal estrogen levels but who do not ovulate, a condition called anovulation. Certain conditions such as low estrogen levels may limit the benefit of clomiphene therapy, especially when not used in conjunction with other assisted reproductive technologies (ART). Women with lower than normal estrogen levels may still conceive by undergoing higher dosages of clomiphene therapy, but I think they would more likely benefit from menotropin therapy, another type of hormone treatment (as talked about earlier).

An important side note, women seeking clomiphene therapy must not have a history of liver disease as the liver metabolizes clomiphene resulting in further damage to the liver. They also should not have any abnormal uterine bleeding, nor any ovarian cysts, as clomiphene may enlarge the cysts.

Physicians usually administer clomiphene between the third and fifth day of menstruation[21] and start with 50 mg per day for a five-day regimen, meaning days five through nine of the menstrual cycle. Ovulation should occur five to ten days after the last dose of clomiphene is administered. If the 50 mg dose is not enough to stimulate ovulation, the physician will increase the dosage by 50 mg each trial until the minimum effective dosage that induces ovulation is reached. (The maximum dosage of clomiphene should not exceed 200–250 mg.) Once that minimum effective dosage is determined, physicians typically recommend the patient undergo four to six treatment cycles at that level until the patient successfully becomes pregnant. During ovulation, the physician instructs patients to have intercourse every other day for one week beginning on the fifth day following the last dose. The recommended dosages have been found effective based on multiple clinical trials. Various methods that determine the exact timing of ovulation are blood tests for luteinizing hormone (LH) levels, urinary tests for LH levels, and ultrasounds to observe the condition of the pelvis.

If the patient is unable to ovulate at the maximum daily dosage of 200–250 mg, the physician may combine clomiphene with other medications such as human chorionic gonadotropin (hCG) or dexamethasone. The addition of hCG to clomiphene therapy may benefit women who respond to clomiphene therapy with rising LH, follicle stimulating hormone (FSH), and estrogen levels but still fail to ovulate. Dexamethasone as an adjunct to clomiphene therapy benefits women with dehydroepiandrosterone sulfate (DHEAS) levels above the normal threshold. DHEAS is a precursor molecule to male and female sex hormones that can increase androgens (male hormones) in the body and result in infertility problems.

Clomiphene citrate causes ovulation by stimulating the pituitary gland to secrete more FSH and LH while stimulating the ovaries to secrete estrogen. After a five-day treatment with clomiphene, LH and FSH levels initially decline but estradiol continues to increase resulting in a preovulatory peak and LH and FSH levels increasing once again.

There are certain risk factors that are associated with clomiphene therapy that should be considered. One is possible luteal phase defect. The luteal phase is the period beginning immediately after the end of ovulation and continuing to the first day of menstruation. During this period, a woman's body normally prepares the endometrium (lining of the uterine wall) for a fertilized egg to implant. However, if there is a defect during this phase, the endometrium is not prepared for implantation. There's also the fact that clomiphene will affect the cervical mucus, which can prevent sperm from entering the uterus and fertilizing the egg.

Most women who undergo fertility treatments first try ovulation induction drugs such as clomiphene before undergoing more expensive procedures such as IVF, which can well exceed $12,000. However, clomiphene therapy does not treat male infertility or female cervical mucus defects, in which case techniques such as IVF are recommended. Unlike most other assisted reproductive technologies, fertility medications such as clomiphene citrate are considered an acceptable fertility treatment by the Catholic Church (as well as other religions), making them the preferred option for some patients.

* * *

Our menstrual cycles trend from proliferation to ovulation to luteal phases and over again. There are so many other finely orchestrated processes going on during our cycle – like hormones ebbing and flowing – that when it doesn't work we tend to look outside of ourselves for answers. The most common remedy prescribed is the oral contraceptive pill (birth control), which comes with a slew of its own problems that range from short acting to lasting for months, even years, once the drug is introduced to your system.

At the end of menses, estradiol production has started to thicken up the endometrium and then, hey presto, you're om the way to starting your cycle all over again, month after month. The lining of the uterus becomes thick until your menses.

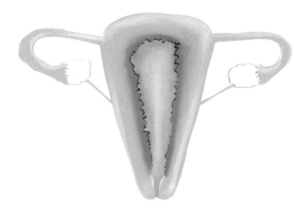

Progesterone production is in full swing and will continue to rise post-ovulation to help support a pregnancy, provided there is one, as well as hold the thickened lining in place. The lining becomes so thick and irritated that soon hormone-like substances (prostaglandins) involved in pain and inflammation trigger the uterine muscle contractions. The higher the levels of prostaglandins, the more likely you are to suffer menstrual cramps, some of which can be severe. Younger ladies in their teens tend to have more prostaglandin so they will complain more of pain during menses. Once the body realizes that it's not pregnant then both hormone levels drop to allow for you to menstruate.

If you're looking to get pregnant, it is usual to start care with an Obstetrician-Gynecologist. The OB-GYN is limited in what she has in her tool bag as far as the extent and depth of care. They are able to initiate lab and ultrasound testing, but most times they send you on your way with Clomid. Many women think that Clomid (Clomiphene Citrate) is the quick and simple solution. While it may work for some, it doesn't always work for many and the side effects can be horrible. Clomiphene tricks the body into producing higher levels of hormones that stimulate the ovarian follicles, causing eggs to ripen and to be released into the fallopian tubes. It was originally thought of as a breast cancer treatment drug because of its anti-estrogenic properties. While treating patients for breast cancers, it was accidentally discovered that the drug also helped induce ovulation.

The standard for the past 40 years is to tell patients that Clomid is the tried-and-true bargain-basement fertility drug to augment natural ovulation in millions of women. They say that it's perfectly safe in one breath, but then in the next they'll say, "Side effects include hot flashes, mood changes, bloating, vaginal dryness, and decreased cervical mucus. Also pay close attention to any visual changes. Black spots in front of the eyes may indicate a more serious side effect. Notify your doctor immediately if you're having issues with your vision."

Over the 20 plus years of my practice I have worked with hundreds of women who've used Clomid and report the same side effects as discussed above. I'll never forget the 37-year-old woman, Anne, with a history of Hashimoto's thyroid[22] using Synthroid[23]. Anne had never been pregnant. She had been trying for one year without success. Irregular menstrual cycles can make it harder for women with Hashimoto's to get pregnant. Studies that I've read show that almost half of women with hypothyroidism due to Hashimoto's disease had problems getting pregnant. Most of these women were recently diagnosed with hypothyroidism or had not yet started treatment for hypothyroidism. Anne's doctor's goal was to get the thyroid as healthy as possible before trying to conceive. TSH is often the only test run for the diagnosis and treatment of thyroid conditions, but this one test does not give a full picture of thyroid health.

*Always insist on a full thyroid panel that includes a TSH, Free T4, Free T3, Reverse T3, Thyroid Peroxidase Antibodies, and Thyroglobulin Antibodies.

I asked Anne to have a new set of thyroid labs done at the start of my work with her. Her TSH was 7 and TPO was 834. Synthroid was not doing its job. In this case there were a few considerations: either the dose was too low or her body was having trouble converting to the active T3 hormone. At this point I asked that she have a reverse T3 blood test. That level was elevated. Synthroid was not the correct course of action for her. I suggested that she start Armour thyroid which is a full spectrum therapy to include T3 and T4. In other words, her thyroid would not have to convert synthetic T4 to the active T3 because she'd already been taking both. Typically, the molecule iodine and Selenium will help with the T4 to

T3 conversion; however, for women with Hashimoto's, the iodine supplement will work in a non-productive manor to produce more antibodies.

For nine months out of the year she'd been trying to conceive using Clomid. Let's keep in mind that I mentioned six side effects and she experienced all of them at some point within that nine-month time span. The maker of Clomid states to not use the drug in a patient that has uncontrolled thyroid disease and not beyond three treatment cycles because it may increase the risk of developing an ovarian tumor and thus decrease one's own natural fertility. At the time that Anne was using Clomid her thyroid antibodies were extremely elevated. In my professional opinion, it was inappropriate to use Clomid in this case. During her numerous medicated cycles she was not being monitored by ultrasound or measuring estradiol to check for good follicular growth. Her doctor would not have known how she was responding to the current dose. However, upon noting that she was not conceiving, her physician kept increasing her medication until she was at a maximum dose.

Anne never did conceive using Clomid; however, she consulted with me to start the Shared Journey Fertility program. The first thing we did was obtain a new thyroid panel which revealed a TSH of 1.9 and a TPO of 80. T3 and T4 were in much better balance and this information comes eight weeks post starting Armour thyroid. Anne ended up conceiving four months after her sixth Merciér Therapy session. Their baby girl was born at 41 weeks at home with the assistance of a midwife.

IN VITRO FERTILIZATION (IVF)

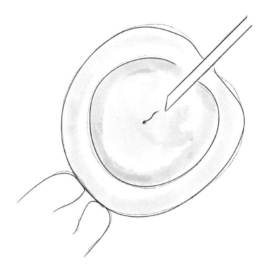

While it is comforting to some to utilize the services of a reproductive endocrinologist, once you do, however, you've attached yourself to an already working machine. You attend your first appointment not knowing what to expect. Once face-to-face with your REI (Reproductive Endocrinology and Infertility), she tells you that *the way* is to monitor one full cycle with labs and ultrasound. She could order a hysterosalpingogram to see if your tubes are open too, and your husband will need to give a semen analysis as well. Once all of these tests and your cycle have completed then you'll convene with your doctor to discuss findings and a treatment plan. This is where the practice of diagnostic medicine ends and the sales pitch begins.

Reproductive medicine is currently an 8-billion-dollar industry in which the most expensive option is offered as the first line treatment to remedy your infertility issues. *The global assisted reproductive technology (ART) market is expected to grow at a*

CAGR (compound annual growth rate) of around 8.6% over the forecast period 2019 to 2026 and expected to reach the market value of around $44.59 billion by 2026 (Acumen Research and Consulting). Keep in mind that more than half of all women with challenges are diagnosed as "unexplained." Unexplained infertility means that there is no answer as to why a pregnancy is not occurring. Yet the machine still believes that they have the answer. All too common, without surprise, that answer is medicine. Intervening medically puts a radically invasive and expensive twist on how you get pregnant.

I always like to point out that one of the most distressing aspects of IVF is its decoupling aspect. Women tend to face the whole juggernaut of IVF treatment alone. They typically attend the appointments alone, inject the medications alone, have the eggs retrieved alone, suffer through the pain alone... and on and on. Maybe your husband shows up for the big embryo transfer day, maybe he offers the very best support, but there will always be the fact that conception happened at the hand of another human. This alone is not the way that we were meant to become pregnant.

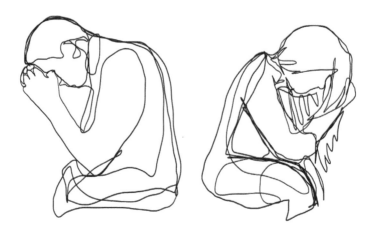

Maybe you feel this in your bones as well, and it is one of the main reasons that brought you to Merciér Therapy. If so, know you first have other options.

However, as previously discussed, I do understand that there are medical reasons that one would need IVF. My main point is that if everything I have discussed is something of concern to you, then you deserve to consider all options at your disposal before you embark on something you may be unsure about. Once nothing else has worked, and you still want a baby more than anything, then IVF certainly is a viable option. However, I would highly recommend – and truly, you owe it to yourself and your precious body – that you explore every other gentler, more nurturing avenue first before harsh medical intervention.

* * *

Usually the first step you'll take in visiting an REI is to go through a basic infertility evaluation cycle to measure baseline lab tests, ultrasound monitoring of follicular growth and ovulation, and possibly a hysterosalpingogram (HSG).

An HSG is when radiographic dye is pushed through the uterine cavity to reveal under x-ray if the fallopian tubes are open. If the tubes are not open, the provider has the option of feeding a guidewire into the tube to remove the blockage or forcing a bit more dye to see if the obstruction will move. I am finding that currently providers are not trying to "unblock" the tubes rather sending women straight into an IVF cycle. IVF is the most successful option for women with non-patent (closed) tubes.

Suppose that you drive halfway over a bridge to discover that the end has a construction closure, and that closure is permanent because the bridge has been deemed a danger. Women with tubal occlusions or past infection usually develop a hydrosalpinx. Hydrosalpinx is a collection of fluid inside of the tube giving the tube a sausage-like appearance. Typically, the cause of tubal damage is a past sexually transmitted infection such as chlamydia, endometriosis, or pelvic inflammatory disease. Tubal narrowing does not necessarily prevent pregnancy, but if pregnancy does occur it may settle into the tube which is how you get an ectopic pregnancy. Ectopic pregnancies are a danger to the woman and usually need immediate medical intervention in the form of medication or surgery to remove the pregnancy.

Sonohystogram is another examination that looks at the cavity of the uterus. Saline is put into the uterus through the cervix using a thin plastic catheter. Sound waves are then used to create images of the lining of the uterus. The fluid helps show more detail than when ultrasound is used alone. In the event that there is pathology present such as a polyp then it is typical to schedule a hysteroscopy to remove tissue that could inhibit implantation.

After that first cycle of monitoring the reproductive endocrinologist will discuss options for moving forward. Ultimately, it will be your decision on what feels best to you. If there is a push toward IVF and that does not sit well with you, then please ask if there are any other options. Usually there are less invasive medically assisted cycles and for whatever reason, these are not often typically discussed, especially if your medical insurance covers IVF.

Who actually needs IVF? Those with blocked tubes, no tubes, non-communicating tubes, possibly some difficult cases of PCOS, and endometriosis. Also Male Factor Infertility requiring testicular extraction, poor overall counts and motility, and morphology issues.

If a large number of fertility cases are unexplained then why are we using such forceful methods to help couples achieve pregnancy? Isn't it best to find the underlying challenge and address that first?

The body is so intelligently designed and it knows exactly what to do if we give it the healthiest conditions to do so. My recommendations are to allow the food to be your medicine by eating nutrient-dense, organic whole foods, utilizing the appropriate supportive supplementation, and possibly assisting your body to become stronger in the luteal phase with implementing bio-identical progesterone.

Changing the oil in a car when it really needs a new tire is defeating the car's ability to operate efficiently. The purpose of the car is to safely transport us from place to place. In other words, the oil is fresh but it remains unsafe to drive. If we decide to proceed, we're likely to create an accident thereby placing ourself or someone else in danger. You catch my drift.

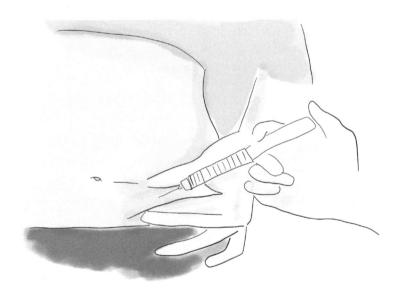

IVF is force. In vitro fertilization artificially manipulates a woman's body to release a multitude of eggs per cycle, retrieving the eggs, and then the embryologist will force the hand-selected sperm into each egg to make an embryo, all of which is very invasive. This process severs innate communication between egg and sperm. In a natural cycle, after the egg is ovulated the sperm will surround the egg and the egg will make the allowance as to what sperm will fertilize the egg. In a fresh transfer cycle, you'll be creating an environment conducive to supporting a pregnancy by utilizing estradiol and progesterone, and that may have long term effects. Around 70% of all IVF cycles do not work. I got this number by loosely averaging the preliminary data for 2019 provided by SART.org. That number is slightly better for women under age 35.

But let's ask the bigger question about why IVF fails so often… In my opinion, and from my experience with women seeking my help, it is clear that the body does not gracefully adjust to being forced. Respecting the natural creation and maturation process of an embryo created within the body is best. If a pregnancy is meant to be, the body is very intelligent and will allow for the process to be near effortless.

If a little medical assistance is needed, my favorite cycle is using an injectable FSH (follicle stimulating hormone) along with an HCG (human chorionic gonadotropin) trigger of ovulation. Sometimes an IUI (intrauterine insemination) is used with kind of cycle as well. I would only suggest the later if there is a male factor issue and advise couples to time their intercourse along with the LH surge (ovulation).

These fertility treatment cycles are often referred to as controlled ovarian stimulation (or hyperstimulation) cycles. Injectable FSH products are also referred to as HMG, human menopausal gonadotropins, or gonadotropins. Brand names for these drugs (hormones) in the

USA include Menopur, Bravelle, Follistim, Gonal-F, and Repronex.

Medications are injected and approximate timing of the monitoring of ovarian stimulation is correlated with the IUI or timed intercourse.

The best time to couple this kind of cycle with an intrauterine insemination is when there is male factor present in the semen analysis. Of all infertility cases, approximately 40–50% is due to "male factor" infertility and as many as 2% of all men will exhibit sub-optimal sperm parameters. It may be one or a combination of low sperm concentration, poor sperm motility, or abnormal morphology.[24]

Should it become necessary to use an IVF cycle then let's get you ready.

First, let's talk about why you might need this protocol. Reasons include blocked or damaged fallopian tubes, male factor infertility including decreased overall counts and motility, ovulation disorders, women who have had their tubes removed, genetic disorder, or unexplained infertility.

So before any treatments, women will have already gone through a testing cycle called the BIE or basic infertility evaluation. An infertility evaluation is usually initiated after one year of regular unprotected intercourse in women under age 35 years and after six months of unprotected intercourse in women age 35 years and older. However, the evaluation may be initiated sooner in women with irregular menstrual cycles or known risk factors for infertility, such as endometriosis, a history of pelvic inflammatory disease, or reproductive tract malformations. Multiple tests have been proposed for evaluation of female infertility. Some of these tests are supported by good evidence, while others are not. Both partners of an infertile couple should be evaluated for factors that could be impairing fertility. The infertility specialist then uses this information to counsel the couple about the possible causes of their infertility and to offer a treatment plan targeted to their specific needs.

A TYPICAL IVF CYCLE MAY LOOK LIKE THIS:

Baseline Test: Day 1

Office visit is scheduled day 2 or day 3 following onset of menses for the purpose of a baseline ultrasound examination and a blood test (usually for follicle stimulating hormone (AMH, FSH, progesterone and estradiol.))

Ovarian Suppression: 2-4 Weeks

Before you start stimulation, they use medication to suppress the ovaries, which can include birth control pills or an injectable medication called Lupron (euprolide acetate for depot suspension)[25]. Lupron in IVF down-regulates the ovaries. During Lupron IVF protocol, the patient starts to receive the injections on the 21st day of the menstrual cycle. The birth control pill puts your ovaries into a temporary state of rest to allow for many other women within your reproductive doctor's practice to undergo the same schedule. This is most efficient for the practice so that all their patients are ready for retrieval and embryo transfer within days of each other.

Ovarian suppression is usually anywhere from 1 to 4 weeks long. At the end of this time, another office visit is scheduled, and an ultrasound and blood test performed to ensure that down-regulation has been achieved. Down-regulation is an important part of IVF treatment which enables the fertility specialist to better control egg maturation and ovulation during the treatment.

Ovarian Stimulation: 8-12 Days

Ovarian stimulation is started with injectable fertility medications on a day that is chosen by the cycle coordinator. A pre-

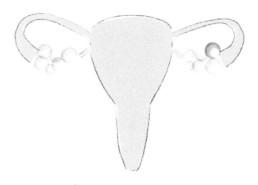

cise dosage of fertility medications (Follistim, Menopur, Gonal-F, Bravelle, Repronex, or a combination of these) per day is begun. Since you may need to change the dose of medication during the day, it is most convenient if the patients take their injections in the evening.

Cycle Monitoring: Starting Day 5

Regular office visits are now begun, starting with day five of stimulation and then continuing every one to two days until follicle aspiration (egg retrieval). During each office visit, an ultrasound and blood test for estradiol are performed.

Ovulation Induction: Between Day 8 and 12

Ovulation is triggered with an injection of human chorionic gonadotropin (hCG), Lupron, or both. Trigger is administered when the follicles are judged to be mature, usually 8 and 12 days after the start of injectable fertility medications. The timing of the hCG dose is very important, because follicle aspiration is performed 36 hours after the hCG.

Egg Retrieval: 36 Hours After hCG

On the day of follicle aspiration, you will be asked to come to the reproductive center and the aspiration procedure itself takes less than 30 minutes.

Sperm Collection: Day of Egg Retrieval

Sperm are obtained from the male partner on the day of egg retrieval. Occasionally, a final specimen may be requested on the morning after egg retrieval if fertilization is sub-optimal and the embryologists have reason to believe that an additional semen specimen would be useful. To optimize sperm quality, it is best to abstain from ejaculation for two to seven days prior to the first sperm specimen. In most cases, this will mean abstinence after the seventh day of fertility medications to the woman.

Fertilization: Day of Egg Retrieval

Sperm are then joined with the eggs to allow fertilization. In most cases, sperm solution is added to the eggs and fertilization occurs naturally. If indicated Intra-Cytoplasmic Sperm Injection (ICSI) will be conducted.

Assisted Hatching

If indicated, Assisted Hatching is conducted to facilitate fertilization. This is routinely done for patients getting preimplantation genetic testing. Assisted Zona Hatching (AZH) is a procedure typically performed on all embryos prior to fresh transfer to the uterus on Day 3-5 of embryo development. This is done to increase the chances of embryo implantation and pregnancy. Each human embryo is surrounded by a "shell" called the zona pellucida. The embryo must break out of this shell for implantation to occur. An unusually thick or hard "shell" is thought to reduce the likelihood of implantation and pregnancy. Therefore, by creating an artificial opening in the shell the likelihood of implantation is thought to increase. Assisted hatching is performed using micromanipulation instruments attached to a microscope. The embryo is held in position by gentle suction from a micropipette. An opening is created in the zona pellucida using a fine glass needle. The needle never meets the embryo but allows for an incision to be made in the outer shell. This procedure is performed in a drop of nutrient medium and afterward the embryo is returned to culture until the embryo transfer procedure is performed. This opening is thought to facilitate hatching (which normally takes place in the uterus) and enhance contact with the lining of the uterus. AZH is most useful for patients older than 38 years of age with elevated levels of follicle stimulating hormone (FSH), or have embryos thicker than normal zona pellucida, or have undergone previous multiple IVF attempts with failed implantations.

Preimplantation Genetic Test: 5-6 Days After Retrieval

If indicated, preimplantation genetic testing (testing for chromosomal status, genetic conditions, and/or gender determination) is done when the embryo is at the blastocyst stage, typically 5-6 days following fertilization.

Embryo Transfer: 3-5 Days After Egg Retrieval

Fresh embryo transfers are done usually 3-5 days after egg retrieval. This is a simple procedure, which does not require anesthesia. Many clinics are now batching embryos while the woman will undergo ovarian stimulation and retrieval all over again.

Excess Embryo Cryopreservation

Any viable embryos more than those transferred back to the patient's uterus may be cryopreserved (frozen) at this time.

Luteal Phase Support: Day of Transfer

You will be given instructions for progesterone supplementation for your embryo transfer. The progesterone is usually administered via injection and vaginal suppositories. Patients are asked to use the progesterone until the end of the first trimester of pregnancy, or when the second blood pregnancy test is negative.

Pregnancy Testing: Day 12 and 14

At least two pregnancy tests are typically done following the embryo transfer. Your clinic will contact you with the results, which are typically available later that afternoon.

This whole process is very long and arduous but well worth it when it ends in a healthy pregnancy.

Each step of the journey provides an amazing lesson and is teaching you more than you could imagine. Choose carefully and from a place of clarity, reason, and understanding. Are you well prepared for your cycle? From an emotional perspective, think about what your ideal cycle would feel like then hang on to that energy.

Our world and all of the people surrounding us will quite possibly give the best multifaceted views of "how to" go about handling life's curve balls. Talk to your friends. Knowledge is power. That is my gift to you. I want you to be as informed as possible so that you can ultimately make the decision that feels best.

* * *

During my many years of practice so many varying stories have crossed my path and some are just tragic and end with fatal consequences to the woman. Ovarian hyperstimulation syndrome (OHSS) is real. Let's discuss it further.

OHSS is an excessive response to taking the medicines (especially injectable gonadotropins) used to make eggs grow. OHSS can result from taking other medications, such as clomiphene citrate or gonadotropin-releasing hormone.

Women with OHSS have a large number of growing follicles along with high estradiol levels. This leads to fluid leaking into the abdomen (belly), which can cause bloating, nausea, and swelling of the abdomen. When OHSS is severe, blood clots, shortness of breath, abdominal pain, dehydration, and vomiting are possible. Rare deaths are reported.

OHSS can be classified as mild, moderate, or severe. One out of three women has symptoms of mild OHSS during controlled ovarian stimulation for in vitro fertilization (IVF). These symptoms may include mild abdominal bloating, nausea, and weight gain due to fluid. Women with moderate OHSS typically have more of these same symptoms. Women with severe OHSS usually have vomiting and cannot keep down liquids. They experience significant discomfort from swelling of the abdomen. They can develop shortness of breath and blood clots can form in the legs.

In all cases of OHSS, the ovaries are enlarged. The size of the ovary is a marker of the degree of OHSS. If symptoms are present, a transvaginal or abdominal ultrasound can be done to measure ovary size and the amount of fluid collected.

Yes, deaths are rare but do occur. I worked for 2 different large reproductive practices during the early 90's and at one of them

I observed a woman with a very high BMI who they allowed to enter an IVF cycle. This woman was 37 with secondary infertility and a BMI of 44. The prevalence of infertility and associated disorders, such as obesity, are on the rise. There were red flags such as hypertension, type 1 diabetes, surgical mesh in her abdomen due to umbilical hernia repair and fibroids. Although the fibroids were intramural (inside the uterine wall) and would not interfere with implantation or carrying a pregnancy.

I remember this woman and her list of drugs before the doctors added five more drugs to that list to include: oral contraceptives, Lupron, Metrodin, Pergonal, hCG and Progesterone in oil.

One morning she came in for monitoring (ultrasound and blood work) and was complaining of a headache. I took her blood pressure with a large cuff as to not skew the numbers and it read 150/100. She had mentioned to me that she had not taken her calcium channel blocker medication that morning. I had this feeling that she was not tolerating her cycle well. By the end of that day her labs revealed her estradiol to be in the 2000s and she had over ten nearly mature follicles bilaterally. I was instructed to have her use 10,000iu of hCG that night and have her egg retrieval a day and a half later.

Her retrieval was uneventful. I cannot remember how many eggs were retrieved and how many of those eggs resulted in an embryo but she did have a transfer on day three. After her transfer she complained of abdominal discomfort and trouble breathing. The RE told her to go to the emergency room where she was evaluated and had six liters of fluid removed out of her belly. This is called ascites. Ascites is an excess of fluid in the peritoneal cavity. The fluid occupies so much space that it pushes up on the diaphragm disallowing for comfortable breathing. Once that fluid is removed then normal breathing typically resumes.

Our patient was released and sent home hours after the fluid removal. The next day she was not feeling well and complaining of a terrible headache again but this time with visual disturbances, floaters in her visual field. The RE told her to go back to the ER to be evaluated. Unfortunately, her husband couldn't get her there quickly enough and she went into cardiac arrest, the paramedics were called, and she died on her way to the hospital. This is an extreme but very real case. In my opinion this woman was far too unwell to undergo an IVF cycle. We have got to be realistic when allowing for women to go into an IVF cycle. Morbid obesity with comorbidities such as hers took her life. I will never forget her. I am really disheartened to see women and couples broken emotionally, financially, and physically due to numerous unsuccessful medicated cycles.

Medically assisted fertility cycles are done far too often. Very heavy doses of superovulation hormones to make multiple eggs verses one per natural cycle must do something adverse to our body over time.

Women typically go through the IVF procedure for three or four cycles before conceiving – or giving up. Some couples make more attempts. There are no regulations limiting the number. No one really knows if IVF hormone treatment plays any role in ovarian cancer, premature menopause, thyroid problems, or other conditions. There are some women who have done up to twenty fresh IVF cycles and were not sure of those longer-term outcomes on individual health.

There have been some studies conducted in the United Kingdom which explains that women who undergo IVF and related procedures are typically exposed to high levels of estradiol, LH, FSH and multiple ovarian punctures, all of which are potentially carcinogenic. There are conflicting and inconsistent results and a lack of information to make a definitive determination as to if these cycles contributed to ovarian, breast, and uterine cancer.[26]

The hormones are taken daily by injection according to a schedule that typically runs 28 days. Side effects can include hot flashes, mood swings, depression, nausea, breast tenderness, swelling or rash at the injection site, abdominal bloating, and slight twinges of abdominal pain. No one really knows that much about the side effects. How effective is the treatment, is not well-documented either. As a result, it is an impossible informed choice.

The American Society of Reproductive Medicine shares in 2015 that serious complications with IVF are rare. However, when Intracytoplasmic Sperm Injection (ICSI) is done along with IVF there may be an increased risk of birth defects. In addition, there is also a slight risk of a chromosomal abnormality with ICSI. That makes sense as an embryologist selects the sperm and injects it directly into the egg. During a natural conception, the egg selects the sperm that it allows to penetrate the zona; therefore hopefully creating a harmonious union, giving the fertilized egg the best chance.

ENDOMETRIOSIS

Let's chat about our magnificent uterus. It is held in place by strong ligaments, and it is remarkably elastic, stretching to about 500 times its pre-pregnancy size. It grows in weight too, from a couple of ounces to more than 2 pounds. When your pregnancy is over, the uterus returns to its original size. Wow!

The function of the ligaments is to support the uterus within the pelvic cavity. The uterosacral ligaments are also bilateral fibrous bands, which attach the cervix to the sacrum. They are also known as the recto-uterine ligaments or sacrocervical ligaments. This supports the uterus and holds it in place.

And the uterus, obviously, is the center stage for our reproductive system. Therefore, it is paramount for fertility to make sure that organ is in its best shape. If something is amiss, if your uterus is not at its healthiest, your odds of getting pregnant can drastically decline.

The most common threat to a woman's uterus is endometriosis.

Endometriosis can be classified into four stages. The American Society of Reproductive Medicine (ASRM) bases these stages on the lesions themselves, particularly the number of endometrial implants and their depth. However, the ASRM revised their classification to include a point system. This point system allows for a way to numerically scale the disease and help determine classification. A score of 15 or less indicates minimal or mild disease. A score of 16 or higher may indicate moderate or severe disease.

*It is important to note that the stage of the disease does not necessarily reflect the level of pain or presence of symptoms.

The stages of endometriosis as classified by the ASRM[27] are:

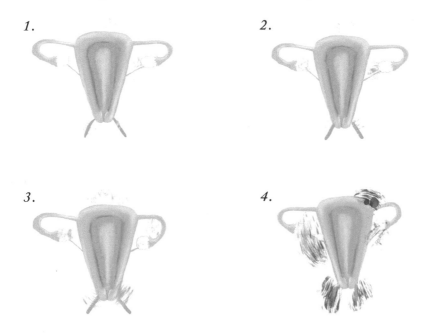

1.

2.

3.

4.

Stage I (1-5 points):

- Minimal

- Few superficial implants

Stage II (6-15 points):

- Mild

- More and deeper implants

Stage III (16-40 points):

- Moderate

- Many deep implants

- Small cysts on one or both ovaries

- Presence of filmy adhesions

Stage IV (>40 points):

- Severe

- Many deep implants

- Large cysts on one or both ovaries

- Many dense adhesions

While these are the official numbered stages of endometriosis as identified by the ASRM, the Endometriosis Foundation of America has proposed using more descriptive categories. This is because every numbered stage has so many variations and does not give any insight into the patient's pain or where lesions can be localized. Therefore, EndoFoundation classifies endometriosis by its anatomical location within the pelvic and abdominal cavity.

The stages of endometriosis as classified by EndoFoundation[28]:

Category I: Peritoneal Endometriosis

The most minimal form of endometriosis in which the peritoneum, the membrane that lines the abdomen, is infiltrated with endometriosis tissue.

Category II: Ovarian Endometriomas (Chocolate Cysts)

Endometriosis that is already established within the ovaries. These forms of ovarian cysts are of particular concern due to their risk of breaking and spreading endometriosis within the pelvic cavity.

Category III: Deep Infiltrating Endometriosis I (DIE I)

The first form of deep infiltrating endometriosis involves organs within the pelvic cavity.

This can include the ovaries, rectum, uterus, and can even lead to such drastic cases as "frozen pelvis."

Category IV: Deep Infiltrating Endometriosis II (DIE II)

The other more extreme form of DIE involves organs both WITHIN and OUTSIDE the pelvic cavity. This can include the bowels, appendix, diaphragm, heart, lungs, and even the brain.

Due to the complex treatment, various anatomical involvement, and expertise and skill that is to be utilized by different surgeons, in other words, for myriad reasons, EndoFoundation prefers to use this descriptive classification system.

So while the symptoms of endometriosis can present itself in the strangest of ways, it can only be officially diagnosed via laparoscopy. If you suspect that you may be suffering from endometriosis, I highly recommend scheduling an appointment with your physician as the disease boasts a very destructive path. Again, symptoms of pelvic pain, ovulation discomfort and bloating, irritable bowels, pain during intercourse and bowel movement, abnormal bleeding, heavy bleeding, and infertility, are all possible signs and should be discussed with your doctor.

As we have already noted, there are many problems that occur with endometriosis and how it pertains to fertility. Chief among them are adhesion formation inside of the fallopian tubes that will block the egg from descending into the tube for fertilization. A good tubal specialist will be able to move a guidewire through the tube and potentially clear the way. Prior to clearing a tube, it can be very helpful to soften up the area to restore movement and blood flow. I have seen an interventional HSG procedure go smoothly after implementing the Merciér Therapy protocol. The easier it is for the physician to perform the procedure the easier it is on the patient.

Chater 4

SOCIETAL AND MEDICAL PRESSURES

Allow me to present a short history of healthcare devices and pharmaceuticals for women.

I'd like to point out the history of some very notable medicines and devices that have been used by women over this last century. All of them were initially deemed safe in humans, but years down the line, we have found out that these items are known to cause major health issues.

Here is a list of a few that I find to be of interest:

PELVIC FLOOR MESH

Pelvic mesh is a woven synthetic netting implanted into the pelvis for a variety of conditions, usually pelvic organ prolapse and stress urinary incontinence. Many women have a good outcome from treatment using mesh; however, some women have experienced harsh complications. Frequently reported complications from transvaginal mesh include chronic pain, infection, bleeding, pain during intercourse, urinary problems, and exposure of the mesh through the vagina. Because this mesh grows into the organs that it supports, it can be very difficult to remove it without damaging the structures. The surgeon must carefully dissect away and repair the adherent organs which leads to unnecessary future surgery.

ESSURE

Essure was a device used for female sterilization. It is a metal coil which when placed into each fallopian tube induces fibrosis and blockage. Essure was designed as an alternative to tubal ligation. Although designed to remain in place for a lifetime, it was approved based on short-term safety studies. In its installation process, two small coils are placed into the uterine horns as a mechanical obstruction of conception. This device was pulled off the market in 2018 due to its terrible side effects, including: back pain, device expulsion and migration, dizziness, fainting, headaches, pelvic cramping, pelvic pain, and vaginal bleeding.

Some women have managed to successfully have them removed without harm to their reproductive organs. Others were not so lucky and had to have salpingectomy (tubal removal) due to tubal damage.

DES OR DIETHYLSTILBESTROL

DES is a man-made (synthetic) form of estrogen. It was pre-scribed to pregnant women between 1940 and 1971 to prevent mis-carriage, premature labor, and related complications of pregnancy. In 1953, published research showed that DES did not prevent miscarriages or premature births. However, DES continued to be prescribed until 1971. In that year, the Food and Drug Admin-istration (FDA) issued a Drug Bulletin advising physicians to stop prescribing DES to pregnant women. "DES Daughters" are defined as women born between 1938 and 1971 who were exposed to DES in utero. Research has confirmed that DES Daughters are at an increased risk for: Clear Cell Adenocarcinoma (CCA), a rare kind of vaginal and cervical cancer. Later it was learned that infants whose mothers took DES during the first five months of pregnancy were more likely to have problems in their reproductive systems, in some cases were even born missing uteruses!

Now, let's look at some other historical facts: for a woman who has an obstruction of a fallopian tube, the procedure of micro-sur-gical connection of tubal adhesions resulted in a 29% "per woman" pregnancy rate even back in the same year the first baby was born as a result of IVF, 1978.

23 years after IVF was first successful, it could muster no more than a 27.5% pregnancy rate, while the success rate with micro-surgery improved.

What about endometriosis? Way back in 1981, women who had received conservative surgical management of this condition had a pregnancy rate of 53%. By 2010, women with this condition using IVF only had a pregnancy rate of 30.8%.

How about polycystic ovaries? Even back in 1950, a "wedge

resection" procedure used by doctors helped women with this condition achieve pregnancy 66% of the time. (This technique now
results in a nearly 80% success rate.) For IVF? Not even 30%. Successful pregnancy rates for artificial insemination are even lower
(less than 20% as acknowledged here by a pro-artificial insemination website).[29]

* * *

One day, I'm sitting at dinner with my children at a lovely local
restaurant and I can't ignore the conversation of the two women sitting at the table next to me. My guess is that these women are in
their late twenties, maybe early thirties. These women are discussing a story about a friend who waited "too long" to have a baby and
had to do IVF. At age 39 she ended up doing four rounds and was
finally pregnant but gave birth early and the baby was in the NICU
for eight weeks but is home now. The one woman went on to say
that this is what happens when you wait too long and the other said
that she will just probably do IVF because she wants to time her
pregnancy and birth.

As I sat trying to play tic-tac-toe with my son, I couldn't
help but think that they knew very little of what they said. I find
that this kind of thinking is sadly commonplace. In 2014, I went
out to film street interviews in Oak Park, Illinois for my documentary and asked ten random strangers what would be the first thing
they'd do if they had trouble conceiving. Nine out of ten said IVF.
After each of them said IVF we stopped filming and I'd ask them
to explain IVF for me. Not one could tell me how it was done and
when I relayed what IVF actually entails, they were shocked. Most

people have no idea the toll IVF takes on a woman's body. From the initial suppression using oral contraceptives and possibly Lupron to stimulation in preparation for super ovulation to egg retrieval to embryo transfer.

I gave birth to my daughter at age 37 and my son at near 41. Older moms are quite exemplary these days. I was reading a current article that states that our natural fertility starts to wane at age 28 and by 35 we just need to hurry up! In general, as a society, women are waiting much later in life to have children than in previous generations. This statistic comes from a variety of reasons, but many women now want to further their career, finish school, have more time with their partner, or simply have not found the right person to couple with. But the pressure, that number 35, looms large and electric always in their brains. It is no wonder that we feel so much pressure.

The time in a woman's life in which she seeks to become pregnant is a season that can be fraught with stress. Basic questions like, when should I start prenatals? Is my diet optimal? What do I need to do to prepare my body? Do I need genetic testing? Can I financially support a child? Am I ready? Those are daunting enough, but throw in fertility issues and the whole thing can feel like the very sky is crushing your lungs.

It is our hope that pregnancy occurs exactly as we plan for it. Does this sound familiar? "I want to be pregnant by February so I can stand up in my sister's wedding and be able to fit into my dress by December" or "I'm a teacher and I'd like to plan my pregnancy and delivery around my summer break." What happens then when there's no pregnancy, and you feel your window of opportunity closing?

When your body throws a wrench into your perfect plans it becomes an all out search to find who can get you pregnant the fastest because, again, plans. In other words, we tend to look for the answer outside of ourselves. This can be dangerous and risky. In our society of convenience where we can literally talk into our smart phone and up comes a list of all options, we have been conditioned into thinking that we can have what we want when we want it. It is tainted on how we view conception as well. Here I am to inform you that God is in charge. He knows exactly when, where, and how your pregnancy will come into existence. It is really comforting to know that we don't have to worry one bit. But we still do worry, a lot, and will literally jump through thousands of hoops to get what we want.

FALSE HOPE

Let us keep in mind the extreme level of hope that a couple has when relinquishing their care over to the reproductive clinic because they sell hopefulness. Women typically disconnect from their own fertility once they have sought out the care of a reproductive endocrinologist and silently bow out of the process because the doctor is now responsible for getting her pregnant. What has actually happened is that she no longer feels responsible for seeking an answer and rather puts all of her hopes into the system to get her pregnant. Not only do we de-couple the couple but medically assisted cycles can drive a wedge into a marriage further, causing longer-term issues.

FORCE

I've always wondered why we force so much on the body. Usually aggression produces a scenario that is unfavorable. I think you are far more likely to acheive your goal by reaching a state of zen calm and accepting what is. (Again, remember our lass with the ladybugs.) Instead of force, first, try giving your body a gentle nudge then allow for a process of healing to occur.

We are constantly making a rush to end in a mad dash. Hurry hurry.

Just one of the definitions for *force* is this (and I believe it to be most appropriate when speaking of medicine): coercion or compulsion, especially with the use of threat. Looking and breaking down the definition further, coercion means the practice of persuading someone to do something by using force or threats. Could we take it a step further and say that threatening the body with invasive means could inflict harm rather than the expected outcome? I would say so.

Let's take a further look at how we force our bodies to outcomes that are exclusively crafted by us.

We actually force the body to have more energy when we drink a cup of caffeinated coffee. I'm guilty of it myself. Taking a sleeping pill is one the more extreme methods of force. My point is, I really want you to think about what happens in your body when you seek out medical care to try to become pregnant. If you have ever been through IVF then you know that this type of cycle is one of the most extreme forces available to you.

Pushing and pushing the body to do what we want it to do can be harmful and especially so if the methods are synthetic. Not to mention that we're unclear of longer-term implications.

Setting out to make good decisions for yourself can be clouded with numerous options. I advise that you do the research on what is available to you with regards to your care. Find reviews of your local community, see what other women are saying. I would advise you also to seek out a local midwife if one is available in your area. Midwives provide a level of care that often obstetricians simply do not have time for. The managed care system limits the amount of time a doctor can spend with her patients. It's really a shame. Midwives have been around much longer than OB-GYNs and, in some countries, (countries with lower infant and maternal mortality rates) they are the norm not the exception. If you live in an area where midwives are not prevalent, you can always hire a doula, someone to help assist you through labor and advocate for you.

Many times, we completely negate our own intuition, cutting us off from our power. Listen to the messages your gut is sending, this is your survival instinct, this is what you feel is the best way deep in your bones. Not listening to intuition can get us in to trouble and makes us think in retrospect about the should haves and could haves, which carry an emotional weight that could have been avoided if you had listened to yourself.

Everything has an expiration (except honey). If you are like most women, you've tried a myriad of modalities to help improve egg quality, normalize cycles, lengthen the luteal phase, reduce cysts on the ovaries, lessen endometriosis pain or chances of miscarriage, clear a blocked tube, or improve your qi etc. Every woman has different circumstances to consider. When on a mission to conceive and carry a healthy pregnancy, all the stops are pulled out and that can lead to a by-any-means-necessary approach. I understand this feeling all too well. Once upon a time I was in the shoes of every woman suffering from infertility, feeling like a caged animal wondering why this was happening to me, exhausted from the stress of the rollercoaster.

My advice is that you choose a gentle method that resonates with you. If you walk away with anything from this book, let that be it. Stick with your decided upon gentle plan for 6-12 months, and then if that doesn't work, move on. If something is not producing the results that you're expecting, it's okay to progress, but my advice is to give it the time it takes. Try not to hurry.

Remember, the definition of insanity is continuing to do something over and over again only to expect that it turns out differently each time. While results may vary from woman to woman this may not yield a pregnancy.

Have you ever focused on something so much that it literally takes over every aspect of your life? Come on now, fess up. I know that you have. We all have. Usually, we can become preoccupied so intently that there's an ability to literally drive us to become sick. By-any-means-necessary behavior can be very dangerous. At any point during our quest, we might feel a mini rumble, an inkling, an intuitive feeling, or an earthquake from within, and sometimes that is enough for us to drop the reigns. Finally, we let go just to take a break. Then a degree of clarity sets in and we decide to maybe change our course and allow the process to unfold with a natural ease.

Because so many women come to me after failed IVF attempts, I've seen this dozens and dozens of times. My goal for this book is to reach some of you *before* you travel down the medically invasive road. I help women at all stages, but if I can save some of you from that unnecessary debilitating process, then I have done my job.

* * *

In the early 1990s I worked for a large reproductive health center. We did the full gamut of medically assisted fertility treatments. While there I was a clinician monitoring cycles, performing semen analysis, Intrauterine Insemination (IUI)[30] and blood draws, assisting with hysterosalpingogram[31], egg retrieval and embryo transfer. It was fascinating and I had especially taken an interest because my plan was to go to medical school then onto an OB-GYN residency and Reproductive Endocrinology and Infertility fellowship.

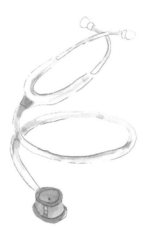

Based on the CDC's 2017 Fertility Clinic Success Rates Report, there were 284,385 Assisted Reproductive Technology (ART)[32] cycles performed at 448 reporting clinics in the United States during 2017, resulting in 68,908 live births (deliveries of one or more living infants) and 78,052 live born infants. Of the 284,385 ART cycles performed, 87,535 were egg or embryo banking cycles in which the intent of the ART cycle was to freeze all resulting eggs or embryos for future ART cycles and for which we would not expect a resulting pregnancy or birth. Although the use of ART is still relatively rare as compared to the potential demand, its use has doubled over the past decade. Today, approximately 1.7% of all infants born in the United States every year are conceived using ART.

While loosely figuring out the numbers as stated above I subtracted the egg and embryo banking cycles from the total of all ART cycles in 2017.

Therefore, 126,942 cycles resulted in no pregnancy.

284,385 (total cycles) - 87,535 (for egg and embryo freezing) = 196,850 - 69,908 (total of live births) = 126,942 (no pregnancy)

I was 35 and desperate to be pregnant yesterday. My husband and I went in to see an REI that I had known for several years. He told us that the only thing for me was IVF. And mind you, this was the second REI that told me that IVF would be the only way. I suspect that due to my diagnosis of severe endometriosis this is the only guidance they could give to me. One went so far as to suggest that I was foolish to not have used Lupron after my last laparoscopy. I did not want to hear that my choice was not what he wanted me to do. Nonetheless, I found myself thinking about using Clomid.

I lost my mind and almost used my arch nemesis Clomid. *Ugh*. Why would I go against my own belief of Clomid being counterintuitive and do something so against my better judgment? I'll tell you why. I felt so broken and needed to do *something*. Clomid felt like the easiest solution for my immediate problem. It is absolutely the most bottom of the barrel drug that depletes women of estradiol which then thins out the endometrium, makes poor fertile mucous, and disallows a hospitable vaginal environment; therefore, most times, requiring an IUI to make it work.

I am so glad that I did not take this awful drug. On top of all that, it would have made me feel more anxious and depressed, more so than what I was already feeling. We opted for unmedicated IUIs. I timed my own luteinizing hormone (LH) surge (ovulation) at home and my then husband and I went into the reproductive endocrinologist for an intrauterine insemination the day after I surged. My husband at the time had a perfect semen analysis, now I know there was no reason to even go this route of IUI.

IUI should be reserved for cases where there is a male factor fertility issue such as poor motility and poor overall counts to help clean up the specimen and weed out all of the sperm that weren't going to fertilize anything. When I worked at the fertility clinic, I performed semen analysis and observed shaky sperm, sperm with flat heads and crimped tails. These as such are a solid reason to get rid of them by washing and preparing the good ones for the big swim ahead. But again, this wasn't the case for us.

Ultimately, I did two home monitored cycles with IUIs, and still, there was not a pregnancy. It became obvious to me that I was not in control. I did note that the signs of ovulation were very consistent. I'd notice fertile mucous on cycle day 12 and 13 then have an LH surge on day 14 or 15. Still, though, no luck.

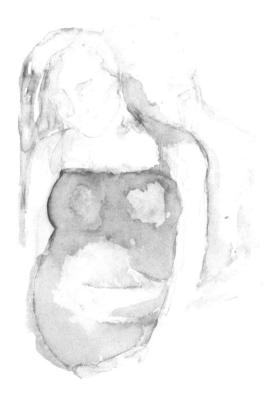

I had my Merciér Therapy students palpate my uterus and ovaries to show me that they knew their maneuvers in class and the next cycle we conceived on our own. I could not believe it!!! It is one thing to have done this for others, it was another to experience it myself. This was the moment I really knew I was onto something. This was when I first conceived a gentle conception.

* * *

I appreciate the reproductive endocrinologists that I work with; they are doing their job, but often lack a practical approach. We need REIs but we also need Merciér Therapy trained professionals. I fully believe that there is a time and place for medicine and also for a gentler, simpler way.

Forcing the body to do something like become pregnant has never sounded so distasteful to me as it does now. After so many years in practice, while observing a multitude of scenarios, I have given a lot of thought to the idea of force. I do not understand what makes us think that force is the best option when helping a couple to become pregnant.

Let us think about this a bit deeper to see what type of emotional, physical, and financial repercussions can come about when someone is not well prepared or well-informed.

My early days spent in the fertility clinic taught me so much. I watched many women fail attempt after medical attempt to try to become pregnant. It was heartbreaking. Some did become pregnant only to miscarry and start assisted cycles all over again.

My heart hurts for all of the couples who put all of their efforts into Western medicine to help them become pregnant. We need to be believing more in ourselves. We are not broken – *you are not broken* – rather, there are probably changes that need to be made to help optimize our own fertile capabilities.

Diet is always the first thing I'd ask a patient to observe. Keep it simple by eating organic foods. I want to observe compliance; making too many changes can feel too overwhelming.

Secondly, did you have an abdominal or pelvic surgical history? And if so did you do any rehabilitation work post operative? Honestly, there aren't many options to aid in recovery. 100% of women are left to their own devices post operatively, to heal on their own with no instruction on managing superficial and deep scar tissue.

A 38-year-old black woman consulted with me and told me her entire medical and gynecological history. Two years prior, she had a laparoscopy that revealed an invasive case of endometriosis. That same day, while she was in recovery, she was rushed back into the operating room because her abdomen was filling up with blood and she was in excruciating pain. The surgeon discovered that her ovarian artery had been nicked and she was bleeding out. Due to the emergent nature of her condition this additional surgery was performed via classical incision (vertical) and she was completely opened for an exploratory view. This second surgery took its toll on her and she ended up needing to be off work for three months. By the time she arrived in my office she was two years post-operative. The scars had turned keloid and underneath was all glued down as if it were frozen in time. She complained of severe intermittent gastrointestinal pain, though anything serious had been ruled out. Her menses came with intense back pain. I did my evaluation to find that her uterus was pulled into an anteflexed position, which was confirmed by ultrasound. Her remaining ovary was very difficult to palpate through the gritty and fibrous connective scar tissue. She then and there committed to my six-session treatment protocol.

I have not had many opportunities to have worked on a belly that was structured like hers. In my opinion this means that women who have this intense scar tissue are not getting the care that they need. With one session to go she reported that her abdominal pain and pelvic tension had been greatly reduced. Though pleased with the outcome thus far, we still had a little more work to go. By the time we finished her last session she was feeling good. Although her goal was to reduce tension in her abdomen and pelvis, she was able to go on to monitor her ovulation cycles and become pregnant naturally at the four-month mark after we finished.

I often wonder why we keep doing the same thing over and over, only to find that the situation never changes. We create human generated problems quite often and rely on "science" to step up to give us the best perspective. I deeply believe that the answer lies within us. It is already there. Does it feel right to you to spend exorbitant amounts of money, time, and emotions on a system that often fails? Could it feel better to invest in your fertility by giving a gentle nudge? Certainly, the force piece is not the best or most gentle. We give our most prized possession away and expect an amazing outcome, yet when we do not get what we expected or needed then we become disappointed, jaded, or enter a state of disbelief.

I think the biggest question is why do we allow our fertility to be handed over to a team to manipulate? I know why: desperation. Why do we become desperate? You probably have been told that you will not get pregnant without their medicine or it'll take a long time so why not just do this right now? Why try on your own any longer when you can simply be rescued by their medicine? After all, we can choose the gender of the baby and genetically test it so that baby is perfect, right? This thinking is not true and presumptive. But we do not have time to investigate further on our own. This era of misinformation is mind-boggling. There is an expected timeline that we are to follow and if it doesn't go as planned then just jump in headfirst to the Western medicine fairyland pool... only to find you're going to hit the ground sprinting.

Desperation leads us to choose the most difficult route to pregnancy possible. I was there when I wanted to be pregnant. After my third laparoscopy I was told that I would not get pregnant without IVF. I knew and felt otherwise but I still listened to those damaging words, which solidified a lack of trust in myself and my body.

I still listened to my intuition, but many, many others listen to the gynecologists when they tell their patients that they will never get pregnant without IVF. It happens every single day and women believe them. Honestly, what gives any human being the right to tell another that something is guaranteed not to be so unless we do this or that? You might say, well, the doctors are trained to know the best way to treat patients because they are doctors. Here is the thing, I've sat in a room full of OB-GYNs and listened to them ask a Reproductive Endocrinologist questions about IVF, and honestly, I thought I was in the Twilight Zone. An astonishing number of gynecologists have no idea what a medically assisted cycle even looks like. I mean, they are not REs, but learning this would seem imperative to a professional suggesting such a practice.

Medically assisted fertility no longer has anything to do with you and your partner and everything to do with appointments, schedules, ultrasounds, blood tests, injections, and procedures. And if all your efforts come to fruition, if that magic formula is compatible with your body, then you'll get pregnant. But what if it does not work? Then what? Most clinics would encourage you to start up your next cycle at the start of your next period. And round and round you go again.

I am here telling you that there is another way.

A woman was once referred to me by a local and very popular reproductive endocrinologist. This patient had already been through having an ovary removed due to a ruptured cyst that ended in infection, was diagnosed with endometriosis, had done numerous rounds of hCG triggered Clomid with IUI cycles and five IVF cycles that ended with four fresh transfers and two frozen embryo transfers (FETs), but none of it ended with a pregnancy. This poor woman went through the proverbial wringer. At this point, she's 42 years old and in my office and completely depleted of eggs, money and emotionally distraught. Why let it get to this dire place? Let's intervene in solid preparation far earlier than the end of the line. Needless to say we did work to let the healing begin and she ended up adopting a sweet little girl.

IVF needs to be reserved for women and men who are in medical need. It is important to remember that the couple may have multiple factors contributing to their infertility. Therefore, a complete initial diagnostic evaluation should be performed to detect or rule out the most common causes of infertility. Ideally, evaluation of both partners is performed concurrently.

Lately I've become more vocal about telling the truth to women. It is my job to talk about our tendency to rush toward options that don't resonate with us but still somehow, we feel pushed or coerced into them. We have got to think about our long-term health as women and as mothers. We have got to think about potential risky family or personal health histories. Let me expand upon this theory.

Most of us are very trusting. We trust that our doctors, physicians, and practitioners are giving us all the information to the best of their knowledge. Some are very trustworthy, others have definitely fudged some details to get you into the most expensive, "easiest" methods. Always do your own research.

When I consult with a couple my intention is to give them the information from my perspective and experience then allow them to make a decision that feels the best to them. No pushing, no coaxing, nothing. I know that my way may not resonate with some and I'm okay with that. Some couples chose medicine first and that's okay. To each their own. I just want you to know that the last stop doesn't necessarily also have to be first. There are other options. It is not up to me to tell anyone what to do, but to present the facts and allow them to decide.

Further exacerbating the pain of infertility for the couple resorting to IVF is the cost. For one round of treatments, a typical out-of-pocket (without insurance coverage) cost is about $14,000. If donor eggs are needed, the cost can easily double or triple. Remember the very low rates of success in getting pregnant after all that, as noted above. How about PGS (preimplantation genetic screening) testing at around $6000 and the possibility of needing the interventional therapy such as IVIG (intravenous immunoglobulin) from a reproductive immunologist? IVIG can cost anywhere from $3500 to $5000 per infusion. But consider the stress this puts the couple under. And, couples with failed IVF treatments (in other words, most of them) are three times more likely to end in divorce.[33]

I was raised Catholic and decided to leave the faith when I was a teenager. It was not feeding me spiritually any longer and I had found great interest in the Evangelical Christian church. I started attending in 1999 and have continued to this day. However, in my opinion the Catholic church makes some valid points that had led me to think deeper on the issues of medical fertility treatments such as IVF.

Nearly 81% of those little babies are never implanted to have the chance to be born. Instead, roughly 250,000 babies conceived from IVF each year are discarded or frozen, and the rate of babies dying in-utero or being selectively aborted is also much higher than with traditional conception. This collateral damage would not seem to be what most of these couples were seeking.[34]

Lately I've been a little hesitant to write for fear of being truthful. I want women to know that there are much more gentler options than to dive headfirst into a shallow, cement-bottomed pond. Please take a look at the statistics yourself and make the best decision based on how you feel. Follow the path of logic when you decide to move forward.

All IVF stats can be located on SART.org which is the Society for Assisted Reproductive Technology. If you decide to move forward into assisted reproductive technology such as IVF then be certain that you are well prepared prior to starting your suppression and stim. There are definitely other options one can try prior to moving into an IVF cycle, such as an FSH injectable, hCG trigger and timed intercourse, or IUI. IUI is or needs to be reserved for cases in which there is male factor present. I was never a big proponent of IUI unless it was medically warranted, plus it does not increase your chances any more than timed intercourse. IUI can drive a wedge between partners if there is an already ongoing emotional issue.

My goal is always to direct a couple to the least overwhelming assisted cycle.

I never want to decouple the couple.

And I always strive to ensure my patients' safety.

I take particular concern with the 60% of women that fall into that nebulous category of "unexplained." Without having an answer, the women in the unexplained category can feel deflated to know that there is no answer medically. I feel that this is a perfect time to clean up the diet, start moving in some type of yoga or Pilates program, **stop** alcohol consumption, **stop** tobacco or any recreational drug use including THC, and limit your caffeine intake. Get your head clear about self-improvement. If you're working with me, I will teach you how to monitor your cycle. We will do this together and you will feel that you've got a proactive partner in your journey. This is the gentle way. You will learn so much about yourself instead of handing it off straight away for a team of humans to manipulate your body and take you further out of the equation of making your baby.

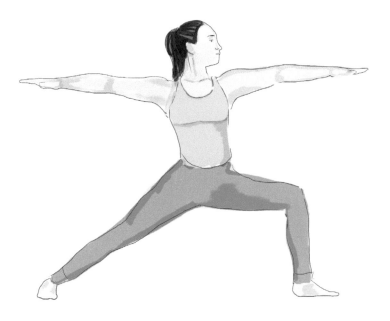

* * *

Pressure from family and friends to have children can be overwhelming. Honestly, I think that these people are well intentioned, but when you're trying to conceive it can be difficult navigating their opinions and questions. Invites to baby showers and baptisms and anything baby-centered may feel like difficult events to attend. Add the targeted ads for baby clothes and it can all be so emotionally overwhelming.

Having a baby is a personal and private choice. If you don't feel like discussing your family growing decisions or fertility issues with friends and family then that is your right. I, however, am an open book and I do feel that by sharing your story, you could not only provoke someone to think differently, but help someone else who may be feeling very alone. When I work with women I always ask them if they're comfortable sharing their fertility journey. Some do want to share and some don't. I respect whichever feels best to that couple. You'll see in the next chapter some women who were kind enough to share their stories with all of you.

Chapter 5

THE SHARED JOURNEY

Becoming free is learning about yourself; the scared and the insecure, the brilliant and the bold. Embrace both and the journey is yours and yours alone. No longer are you following another's directions and your path and purpose will present themselves. Only then might you find another wandering soul doing the same thing, who can walk with you but on their own journey. All of a sudden you might find a shared passion and a wrinkled map on the trail that makes sense.

RIITTA KLINT, ARTIST

When we establish human connections within the context of shared experience we create community wherever we go.

GINA GREENLEE, *POSTCARDS AND PEARLS: LIFE LESSONS FROM SOLO MOMENTS ON THE ROAD*

E very one of these stories is from a patient or former patient of mine. They all have been gracious enough to lend me their stories in the hope that they will offer someone going through something similar some hope and encouragement. You are not alone in your fertility issues. You do not have to live in a world where no one understands or advocates for your health. We at Merciér Therapy care very deeply about every one of our patients. We cheer every time – every single time – we see your positive pregnancy test results. My office is pasted with pictures of all the healthy babies we have helped bring into this world and each one of them fills my heart up with joy.

I want to take this space to thank these people for allowing me to share their harrowing stories with you. They expected a miracle and God delivered.

Please note, some of the names have been changed to protect my clients' identities.

Cynthia

Cynthia and her husband Rich are both Emergency Room Physicians. In her late thirties she wanted to try Merciér Therapy before attempting any medically assisted options. We did our work together and because time was of the essence, I sent her off to a reproductive endocrinologist. I asked the RE to consider an injectable FSH, hCG trigger, and timed intercourse cycle. The patient and the RE discussed it and determined that they would try this first. In just her first stimulated cycle she made one glorious and juicy follicle which became a healthy pregnancy. After nine months, she delivered a healthy baby girl.

Very shortly after her daughter was born, she wanted to start trying for a second child. At that time, she was 41. She ended up doing two fresh IVFs with the same RE that monitored her first less invasive cycle. Both IVFs ended in day three transfers and neither produced a pregnancy.

Her and I talked about it, and she decided to switch to a different practice. I sat in on the consult and the plan was for her to try a new IVF protocol. She ended up doing three more IVF cycles and by the time the third cycle ended she was 43. All three cycles she did fresh transfers on day 3, though none of them produced a pregnancy. The patient decided to give it a rest and not pursue any additional cycles.

Three months after finishing her last round she was feeling extreme fatigue to the point she was struggling to think clearly while seeing patients. Her weight loss was significant. She decided to consult with a medical endocrinologist to run the gamut of tests. All the tests came back to reveal adrenal insufficiency, which is a condition where the adrenal glands do not produce adequate amounts of steroid hormones, primarily cortisol, but may also include impaired production of aldosterone (a mineralocorticoid), which regulates sodium conservation, potassium secretion, and water retention.

In layman's terms, no cortisol equals death. She now injects cortisol twice weekly and feels better, yet her body is still in a state of ups and downs.

I fully believe that the last three IVF cycles threw her into a tailspin causing the endocrine trouble from which she now suffers. The hormones must remain somewhat in balance for the entire dance to be flawless.

This is all further evidence that when we pound a thumbtack with a sledgehammer, it's a cocktail for disaster.

Esther

Esther, age 39, had a history of four laparoscopies to clear up varying issues due to stage 3 endometriosis. She has never been pregnant. Her first laparoscopy was done to explore for endometriosis and confirm the diagnosis. There was nothing significant noted at that time except some powder burn marks on the uterine surface. The second surgery was done to figure out the source of her right-sided pelvic pain. Turns out that she had adhesions which pulled her ovary directly behind her uterus. The third laparoscopy was done due to deep pelvic pain with intercourse and this time it was discovered that both ovaries had migrated to the back of her uterus and were stuck in place. The fourth surgery was also done due to pelvic pain and severely painful menstrual cramping. This had revealed adhesions in the rectouterine pouch and a sizeable endometrioma on the right ovary. All the while she was having unprotected intercourse and did not become pregnant.

Our first visit consisted of me taking Esther's entire history and performing a pelvic organ mobility evaluation. Upon palpation she guarded a lot and complained of mild to severe discomfort throughout her abdomen and pelvis. Each subsequent surgery bears consequences concerning the level of scar tissue produced as aftermath.

I discovered that her uterus was in an anteflexed position and most likely adherent to her bladder. It was very challenging to feel her ovaries, probably because they had migrated to the back of her uterus as verified by pelvic ultrasound. This is called kissing ovaries, an adorable name for a deplorable situation. I had also experienced this personally. My theory is that if there is severe organ misalignment and decreased movement, then blood flow is constricted, causing poor overall organ function. Medicine has no solution nor do they pay any attention to the probability of how this might affect a woman's fertility.

We got to work and she reported that four days after the first session her menses started and that she had never experienced such a pleasant menstrual cycle. Her pain level went from debilitating to tolerable and instead of using many pain-reducing, over-the-counter drugs, she was able to manage with virtually nothing. This kind of change is tangible and promising.

Keep in mind that endometriosis is very aggressive, so while her pain might be at bay in the interim, it would assuredly return.

We kept on working and finished our sessions. At the end of our manual work together I put Esther on an inflammatory reducing protocol and asked her to keep track of her cycles. The supplements and bio-identical hormones that we used to get her feeling well were all safe with pregnancy.

At a three month follow up visit I could see that she was recording good quality fertile mucous and LH (lutenizing hormone) surges around the 12th day of her cycle.

Month four, post treatment completion, Esther called me with a positive pregnancy test. At age 40 she went on to have a non-eventful 38 week pregnancy and vaginally delivered a healthy baby boy.

We do maintenance treatments to help keep her menstrual pain at bay and this has seemed to work very well without the use of harmful drugs or procedures.

Serena and Joe

There's a lot to be said for keeping a couple together during the time that they navigate their way through a fertility challenge. I've seen otherwise and it really can weaken a marriage.

Joe and Serena came to visit me and it was very clear that they were divided on where they stood concerning IVF. I am always especially delighted when husbands come in with their wives. This is the first step toward including both partners in the process. Initially, I noticed Joe reaching for his wife's hand and her reluctantly holding his. I asked them if everything was okay and he mentioned that they had been arguing on the way to my office. I asked them if I may know the reason and they shared that Serena was dead set on doing IVF the following cycle and that he wanted her to work with me first. I explained to them both that I would take their history, perform a pelvic organ mobility evaluation, and give them both my opinion as to how I would approach their fertility challenge. Seeing the look on her face I told her that I do not blow smoke and that honesty will be a part of my delivery.

Serena and Joe were in their early thirties. Joe worked in IT. He had a normal semen analysis, was a non-smoker and was in very good overall health. Serena works as a family law attorney and had an uneventful medical history, only having her tonsils removed at age six. I always ask what someone does for a living because I want to know if they're handling volatile chemicals. So I went on interviewing to find that her AMH[35] (anti-mullerian) is 2.4 and her cycle day 3 FSH is 7.

Menstrual cycles are every 28 days like clockwork. She had a fair amount of cramping and discomfort on the first day of her cycle. She told me: "The pain goes into my lower back and down the front of my legs. I have to take loads of Ibuprofen during the early part of my cycle. The pain finally subsides and I am able to rest but I'm not able to go into work the first day of bleeding."

I asked her if she felt pain during any other part of her cycle such as during ovulation. She said no. How about pain with intercourse or bowel movement? She said yes to both. Without having a diagnosis of endometriosis her pain patterns sounded a lot like there is disease in her pelvis and abdomen. Serena had never been pregnant and becomes emotional upon telling me. No surgery? Abnormal PAP smears? Headaches? Breast tenderness?

"We've tried on our own for ten months and no pregnancy!"

Joe and Serena fall into the 60% of the "unexplained" infertility category, yet first she pursued the medically assisted fertility route and had four failed cycles under her belt. You see, despite there being a normal semen analysis, bilateral tubal patency, normal saline sonogram, nary a thyroid issue, positive signs of ovulation, and an LH surge, she still thought that someone else had all the answers for her.

Serena explained to me that she had done three cycles of Clomid and one cycle of Letrozole. Remember, Clomid is estradiol inhibiting and causes a thinner than normal uterine lining, poor fertile mucous and a hostile vaginal environment. Clomid works by making the body think that your estrogen levels are lower than they are, which causes the pituitary gland to increase secretion of follicle stimulating hormone, or FSH, and luteinizing hormone, or LH.

Serena committed to working with me. We completed our

Mercier Therapy sessions, I put together a supportive supplemental protocol for her and taught her how I wanted her to monitor her cycles. She went on her way and had many questions as she checked in often. It was really neat to hear from her so often as she would be excited to notice that she was ovulating consistently and had all the signs of a healthy cycle. With each passing cycle she would notice new things such as adjustment in cycle length, better quality fertile mucous and a noticeable temperature spike right after ovulating. These are all things that she was missing prior as her cycles were being monitored by a team. She was feeling good now as she had taken her own fertility back. I give every woman a journal in which to record their cycles and encourage writing beyond just cycle notes. Serena had one of the most beautiful journals as she would use colored pencils to illustrate how she was feeling and noting changes. The change in her was remarkable. We checked in at the 5-month post therapy cycle and realized that she was on the 34th day of her normally 28 day cycle. I asked her to go to the pharmacy and pick up a pregnancy test, bring it back to my office and test. She gladly went on her way to arrive back and take the test which turned out to be positive. I was elated for her. She was in shock! We stared at the test together and she cried. It was a beautiful moment and one that I will never forget. Serena and Joe selected a local obstetrician and at 41 weeks vaginally delivered a baby boy. This couple has since come back to visit me for three additional rounds of Mercier Therapy and each time they conceived on their own. They now have four children and are like family to me. I am grateful that Serena gave me a chance to help her and believed that she was not broken.

Joanne and John

I first met Joanne and John, both 34, after they had failed 2 Clomid/intrauterine insemination cycles and two fresh IVF attempts. While taking Joanne's history I asked her for the details of her assisted cycles. She brought her newest cycle day 3 labs which revealed an AMH of .8 and FSH of 9. I knew already that her ovarian reserves were diminished, but there was no pelvic surgical history, which is great and tells me that there is minimal scar tissue present. However, Joanne had undergone two egg retrievals.

Scar tissue refers to thick, fibrous tissues that corrodes healthy tissue; this often happens from a cut, significant injury, or after surgery. Tissue damage may also be internal, so scar tissue can form post-surgery or because of disease. The nature of scar tissue can cause the associated organs and tissues to become glued in place; hence reducing optimal organ movement, blood flow and overall function.

An egg retrieval can commonly cause mild internal bleeding and the potential for scar tissue formation around the ovaries and fallopian tubes. Egg donors are routinely told this could interfere with future natural conception by preventing an otherwise normal egg from entering the fallopian tube after ovulation.

From here, we started our work together. I learned that John had a normal semen analysis and wasn't a smoker. Joanne's tubes were open bilaterally and she lived a healthy lifestyle. As we worked through her six Merciér Therapy sessions we would talk about the cycles they had done leading up to meeting me. Joanne would talk with me about the differences of her IVF cycles as she worked with two different clinics.

I am familiar with both clinics. The first clinic that she worked with was staunch on telling her (and all their patients) that no outside holistic approach has been proven to help. The second clinic gladly supported whatever this couple wanted to try. I really appreciate the collaboration of minds to bring the best results for this sweet couple.

Joanne and John arrived for their last session and I went over their supportive supplement regime. I taught her how to monitor her cycle at home. As you've been reading, the Shared Journey Fertility program concludes with me giving a journal in which to record the details of her cycle. I know that there are many apps out there that record a menstrual cycle for you; however, I think that putting pen to paper actually ignites creativity, inspiring optimism, whereas a phone is more likely to cause stress and negativity. Joanne agreed to give herself a few months of rest from the rigors of IVF. During this time the couple strengthened their marriage and were ready to endure IVF again.

Her first IVF cycle back (really her third cycle) after going through the Merciér protocol helped with a solid stimulation cycle which yielded more eggs than she'd ever had in prior cycles. Joanne had their one and only embryo freshly transferred on day 5. On that day the embryo had grown to a blastocycst. A blastocyst is an embryo which has been left to develop until day 5 or 6 and presents a complex cellular structure formed by approximately 200 cells. The blastocyst phase is the development stage prior to implantation of the embryo in the woman's uterus.

Blastocyst transfers have a higher pregnancy rate than embryos transferred at an earlier stage.

This IVF cycle post Merciér resulted in a pregnancy. Joanne

carried this pregnancy until 9 weeks when the fetal heart rate stopped. It was suggested that she have a D&C to remove the pregnancy. She came in and we worked a one-hour Merciér session to try to initiate the process of a natural miscarriage. The miscarriage occurred in a timely manner and uneventfully.

Joanne gave herself an eight-week break and wanted to try one last fresh IVF cycle. Once again she stimmed very well to end the cycle with one viable embryo, which was also transferred at the blastocyst stage. This cycle resulted in a healthy pregnancy. This couple welcomed a healthy daughter and are very happy.

Caroline and Will

Caroline and Will set up an appointment to discuss their struggle with secondary infertility. As an established patient, I have known Caroline for many years. She had a laparoscopy done at age 28 to determine that she has stage 4 endometriosis. This disease has pained her for many years and now she has a definitive reason for her immense suffering. We worked together on managing her pain several years ago and now she's returned to help improve her fertility. While updating her history there are a couple of things that I noted which could be contributing to her ill luck in trying to conceive for a second time.

First, she had to have a second laparoscopy to help remove endometrial adhesions. Also, her thyroid was under functioning. The reproductive endocrinologist asked her to start taking a small dose of levothyroxine. Caroline's tubes were bilaterally clear and open and Will had a normal semen analysis. Her cycle day 3 FSH is 22.9. This alone makes her a poor candidate for IVF as she was already making too much FSH and would probably not stimulate well.

Thus far her history with endometriosis wasn't unusual from what I've seen in the past but she also had a significant diminish in her ovarian reserve.

Five months prior to seeing me she had consulted with a reproductive endocrinologist. He is a well known physician who was an expert in endometriosis surgery. She felt that she was in good and capable hands. That doctor recommended that the couple proceed with a Clomid cycle. Caroline explained to me that she was prescribed Clomid 100mg to use on cycle days 5-9.

It appeared that she stimulated well on the medication and grew two decently sized follicles during her cycle. She did ovulate as confirmed by ultrasound though this cycle did not produce a pregnancy. After this cycle completed she sat down with the reproductive doctor and he recommended that she proceed forward into an IVF cycle. The couple was not ready to go into an IVF cycle and decided to return to me for my opinion.

I did a pelvic organ mobility evaluation and found that her uterus was restricted in its anterior to posterior movement. This means that her uterus was not easily moved when pressure was applied via the abdomen. When I feel a restriction such as this, I know that the endometriosis is busy at work gluing everything in place. I also know that the blood flow to her organs wasn't as optimal as it could be. Blood flow is the essence of organ health and function.

Based on all of her information I recommended the Shared Journey Fertility program. One month later she started working with me. Her sessions were uneventful and pleasant, relieving pelvic pain in the interim.

At the end of her Merciér Therapy sessions I started her on the diminished ovarian reserve protocol to include DHEA 75mg each day continuously. I gave her some other supportive supplements for her thyroid. We went over how I wanted her to monitor her ovulatory cycles on her own. I gave her the journal to help guide her to keep track of her cervical mucous, LH surge, and timing of intercourse.

After four months of working with me, Caroline had a positive pregnancy test. Her pregnancy was uneventful and they are thrilled to have a son.

Kate and Tim

After trying to conceive for 16 months, Tim and Kate came in for a fertility consultation. While gathering her information Kate explained that they had done four Clomid and intrauterine insemination cycles with no success.

Her gynecologist performed a hysterosalpingogram (HSG) to reveal that both of Kate's tubes were patent (open). Tim had a semen analysis which showed that he had a decrease in motility or the inability of the sperm to move independently. Once the gynecologist had finished her work-up she referred the couple to a reproductive endocrinologist.

A basic infertility evaluation is typically the place where they will start to gather all of the data from one monitored cycle. Let us break this down...

Ovarian Reserve tests are done typically on cycle day 3 of the menstrual cycle.

AMH (anti-mullerian hormone) is a hormone secreted by cells in developing egg sacs (follicles). Remember, the level of AMH in a woman's blood is generally a good indicator of her ovarian reserve. AMH does not change during the menstrual cycle, so the blood sample can be taken at any time of the month – even while you are using oral contraception.

FSH (follicle stimulating hormone) is an important part of the reproductive system. It is responsible for the growth of ovarian follicles. Follicles produce estrogen and progesterone in the ovaries and help maintain the menstrual cycles in women. The level of FSH found in the blood on cycle day 3 can help to predict what the egg reserve is like.

Estradiol level on day 3 (we do it on any day between days 2 and 4) of the menstrual cycle is a way to potentially discover some of those women with a normal day 3 FSH that may in fact have decreased egg quantity and quality.

The LH blood test measures the amount of luteinizing hormone, which is also secreted by the pituitary gland. In women, LH levels rise at mid-cycle; within 24 to 36 hours, ovulation occurs. Higher-than-normal levels of LH can indicate several disorders, including ovarian failure and polycystic ovary disease.

Intravaginal gynecologic ultrasound is used to assess follicular growth throughout the cycle. It would be usual to have an ultrasound on your cycle day 3 to check the antral follicle count. This count is significant and measures a woman's ovarian reserve, or her remaining egg supply. The ovarian reserve reflects the fertility potential.

Pelvic ultrasound is also performed on day 21 to see if ovulation occurred. This imaging would show a corpus luteum cyst and along with the post ovulation scan would be a progesterone blood level. Combined, these two tests will show if ovulation actually occurred.

Kate reconvened with her REI to discuss a plan for moving forward. Her FSH level at 33 and AMH level at .24 suggested a diminish in ovarian reserve. One study concluded that very low AMH levels are associated with a relevant risk of cycle cancellation. In other words, if a woman is making too much FSH against a very low AMH level then there may not be enough FSH to give to be able to effectively stimulate egg production. In vitro fertilization was recommended, and all of her drugs were ordered. The couple weren't quite ready for IVF so they decided to try the Shared Journey Fertility program first.

During our work, Kate would notice that she felt more of an invigorating and open feeling within her pelvis. I put her on a few supportive supplements, and we finished our work together in September. She monitored her ovulation at home for the months of October and November. December rolled around and Kate missed her menses, so she took a home pregnancy test. Kate was pregnant and went along to deliver a healthy baby girl.

Given the result of Kate's ovarian reserve tests, conceiving in short order with her own egg is just another one of those incredible miracles!

Heather and Jonathan

I met a couple who were sent to me through a friend. Heather and Jonathan came to me after they'd been married for 11 years without one successful pregnancy. Upon taking her history, I noticed that she had very normal 28 to 33 day menstrual cycles with a slight bit of cramping on the first day. A hysterosalpingogram was performed to determine that both of her tubes are bilaterally patent (open) and a laparoscopy done to further evaluate what the problem could be.

The laparoscopy had revealed a slight bit of endometriosis, certainly not enough to be a real concern. As we delved deeper into her gynecologic history, I learned that Heather and Jonathan had tried three cycles of Clomid with intrauterine insemination. These were monitored cycles. Heather would receive ultrasound exams concurrent with the use of the drug. This was to make sure that she was not overstimulating and growing a decent follicle per cycle. Once a follicle is measuring 18-20mm it's time to trigger ovulation and perform IUI. Jonathan had a normal semen analysis. All three cycles resulted in a negative pregnancy test.

They decided to continue trying to conceive on their own. In the meantime, they adopted three little boys.

I noticed that Heather's color in her cheeks and lips were quite pale so we checked her hemoglobin. The hemoglobin is a protein component of red blood cells that carry oxygen to all other cells and organs. Heather had a hemoglobin level of 10 and normal levels are 12-16. Once pregnant, the reserve of hemoglobin lowers due to hemodilution. I started her on a food-based iron which could be easily tolerated and told her we would recheck her level in four weeks. Miraculously, her Hgb came up to 14.2! With her next menses the level came down to 12 and remained there.

I always feel that there could be puzzle pieces missing when caring for a woman. There is a level of astonishment when reviewing medical records and wondering why it looked incomplete. I notice quite often that exams and tests have gone undone and wonder why. I never want to leave any stone unturned as this could be the missing piece that weaves the entire picture together.

We got to work. I performed six sessions of Merciér Therapy on Heather over six weeks. She never complained of any pain or tenderness after our sessions. At the end of the six weeks I had put together a customized supportive supplement and bio-identical hormone protocol and asked her to monitor her cycles for LH surge. Heather was no stranger to cycle monitoring. I gave her the journal that I give to all women who finish their sessions. Within the journal is a spot for each day of the cycle to record for the LH surge, the consistency and appearance of cervical mucous, any additional symptoms such as breast tenderness or headaches and when they have intercourse. I love when women take charge of monitoring their own cycles. It creates a sense of being pro-active and in partnership with me.

Heather would check in with me from time to time to let me know how monitoring was going. I asked her if she could see any consistencies or inconsistencies within her cycles. She was noticing very regular surge patterns with an abundance of fertile mucous. Intercourse was timed perfectly and by the 6th cycle Heather and Jonathan had a positive pregnancy test. They were elated and in disbelief. This was a sight that they had never seen before. For me to receive this news is the best thing in the whole world! To be completely honest, I was praying that this couple would be blessed sooner rather than later as they had waited so long.

Baby girl, Jubilee, was born into a loving family of three big brothers. Heather and Jonathan went on to have two more beautiful baby daughters via natural conception. They always joke with me saying that Merciér Therapy is the gift that keeps on giving. I could not be more pleased.

Mandy

Mandy, age 37, consulted with me about the pelvic pain that she had been experiencing. During her visit I learned that she had two natural conceptions and both babies were born vaginally.

The pain that she described was a stabbing and sometimes shooting pain in her deep middle pelvis. She complained of pain with bowel movement and intercourse. There was random sharpness on any given day and sometimes it forced her to call off her whole day. Upon taking her history, she revealed to me that she had the Essure placed in her uterus at age 34. Essure was a device on the market for female sterilization. It is a metal, spring-like, coil which when placed into each uterine horn induces fibrosis (scarring) and blockage.

If you've ever unscrewed a ball-point pen then you've probably seen the small metal spring coil that allows for the pen to retreat into the pen tube and again to release the pen to write. This is exactly what the Essure looks like.

Essure was designed as an alternative to tubal ligation. Although designed to remain in place for a lifetime, it was approved based on short-term safety studies. In years to follow, the many women who received this device started to complain of pelvic and abdominal pain. I asked her if she recalled the exact time frame that her pain started. Mandy mentioned that she started noticing a sharp sensation about four months after having the Essure placed. I asked her if she had the placement of the device checked with a pelvic ultrasound. She said that she had not had an ultrasound done. It wasn't until the documentary film, *The Bleeding Edge,* was released on Netflix that she deduced her pain could be possibly related to the Essure device. I advised her to make an appointment with her gynecologist just to be sure that the device was correctly placed.

Merciér Therapy cannot be used when there is any device such as Essure, IUD, or tubal clips. Our deep visceral application sequence could potentially disrupt the placement of the latter and cause perforation of surrounding structures.

After Mandy's appointment with her gynecologist and her ultrasound was completed, she came back in to discuss the findings. The ultrasound report revealed that the Essure coils started to break down in both of her uterine horns and some of the coil on the right side was missing. Any foreign object floating around inside of the body has the ability to perforate tissue, causing pain, bleeding and possibly infection.

My next suggestion was to seek out a surgeon to have this device removed so we could start our work together.

Mandy found a surgeon in California that was removing many Essure devices and promptly scheduled her removal surgery.

I advised her to come back and see me when she was six weeks out of surgery. With her surgeon's clearance, we started our work together to start to heal the scarring in her tubes. After the first visit she felt immense relief and was able to successfully be intimate with her husband and achieve orgasm without pain. I was so pleased to hear this as she had explained to me that it was years since she was able to have pleasurable sex without the fear of pain. Her husband was thrilled to be creating a renewal within their marriage and they became closer.

After completing six Merciér Therapy sessions I told her to let me know if she needed more work and that I also wanted a full report moving forward. It was only three months after we finished that she called to tell me that they were expecting their third baby! This pregnancy was a complete and awesome surprise.

Mandy and Dave welcomed their son, born uneventfully via vaginal delivery.

Heather and Tim

With a referral from a friend in Illinois, Heather and Tim travelled from Texas for the Shared Journey Fertility program. They figured, *why not?* as their Illinois friends had success shortly after finishing the work with me.

Upon taking Heather's history I took note of her current numerous prescribed meds: Metformin, Spironolactone, Sertraline, Topamax, Promethazine (category C), and Maxalt (a migraine medication that is a category B1 which means not adequately tested to deem 100% safe in pregnancy). The first four meds listed are category B which means that those drugs have been well studied and deemed safe in pregnancy.

Heather told me that she was occasionally suffering from migraine headaches and the medications were helping somewhat to keep them at bay. Also notable is her diagnosis of polycystic ovary syndrome, or PCOS. She explained to me her lengthy cycles accompanied by a ten day painful menses. On occasion she had experienced discomfort from ruptured ovarian cysts.

Here's the thing: with elevated male androgen hormones such as DHEA and testosterone this alone can cause headaches. Her primary doctor suggested that she may be suffering from migraines; hence the medication regime. Most women with elevated androgen levels have PCOS.

That said, there are other possible causes of hyperandrogenism and the list of hormones below must be taken into account as well.

- Androstenedione (A4)

- Androstenediol (A5)

- Androsterone

- Dihydrotestosterone (DHT)

There are two "kinds" of hyperandrogenism: clinical and biochemical. Having either type may qualify a woman as having PCOS. Clinical hyperandrogenism is when there are visible signs or symptoms that indicate that androgen production may be higher than expected. These are things that can be seen or experienced without medical testing. Biochemical hyperandrogenism is when lab work shows abnormally high levels of androgen hormones in the bloodstream.

Some of the symptoms of PCOS are: abnormal hair growth on the face, chest, or back. Note, this is hair growth usually associated with men, like facial hair or chest hair, and can be a clinical sign of hyperandrogenism. The medical term for this is hirsutism. Between 75 and 80 percent of women with male-like hair growth have PCOS, but not all women with PCOS experience this symptom. Many women remove this excess hair growth and may not realize it is a potential symptom of a medical problem. (Be sure to tell your doctor if you are experiencing hirsutism.)

Acne is another symptom. Acne during adolescence is common in teenagers, both boys and girls. Even in adulthood, mild acne is not considered to be abnormal. However, moderate to severe acne, especially when accompanied by other troublesome symptoms, can be an indicator of excess androgens.

Male pattern balding as well. Both men and women may experience hair loss as they age. However, when women experience "male pattern balding," especially at a younger age than might be expected, this can be a possible sign of clinical hyperandrogenism.

Virilization too. This is when a woman develops traits associated with men, like a deepening voice or more male-like muscle growth. While this is a possible clinical sign of hyperandrogenism, it is not usually seen with PCOS. Other possible causes of hyperandrogenism should be considered.

Biochemical hyperandrogenism is when blood work indicates that androgen levels are higher than normal. Testing androgen levels when making a diagnosis of PCOS is important. Even if there are clinical signs of hyperandrogenism already evident, blood work can help rule out other possible causes of hyperandrogenism.

Below are the androgens that may be tested and what levels are normal. The normal ranges may vary with the lab.

NORMAL RANGES OF ANDROGENS

Total testosterone: Levels should be between 6.0 and 86 ng per dl in women. In PCOS, total testosterone may be slightly elevated. Extremely high levels of total testosterone may indicate an androgen-secreting tumor.

Free testosterone: Normal levels of free testosterone are between 0.7 and 3.6 pg per mL. Free testosterone levels may be elevated in PCOS.

Androstenedione: Normal levels in women are between 0.7 to 3.1 ng per mL. Elevated levels may indicate PCOS.

DHEA-S: Normal levels in women are between 35 and 430 ug/dl. Women with PCOS may have levels over 200, which fall within the normal but high range. Extremely high levels of DHEA-S may indicate an androgen-secreting tumor.

Back to Heather's history: as she monitored her own cycles she didn't necessarily notice consistent ovulation indications such as mucous or LH surge. This is pretty typical with PCOS.

Heather came to me in 2016 seeking Merciér Therapy. Her history of fertility treatments started in 2010 and included Clomid 50mg used on cycle days 3-7. She did not grow a follicle according to the mid cycle ultrasound and this cycle resulted in no pregnancy. At the time they decided to not pursue any additional cycles. It took three more for them to want to try again. They used Femara for two cycles with an hCG trigger of ovulation and timed intercourse. Tim had a normal semen analysis. But both cycles resulted in a negative pregnancy test.

As a side note, I'm very glad they never pursued IVF as another nasty side effect can be increased headaches, in both frequency and severity.

We got to work and applied 90 minutes of Merciér Therapy each day for four days. Heather tolerated her sessions very well and explained to me each day after her session that she was very fatigued. This is normal and I have observed it with many women. There is a large network of lymphatic glands in the pelvis and when I apply my work with its depth it will move that lymphatic fluid causing a toxicity that needs to be excreted. This alone can cause fatigue. I am really pleased that she was able to rest.

During our time we discussed her discontinuing some of her medications with her doctor. She was on board and moved forward to stop the Spironolactone and Topamax. As it was clear to me and Heather that neither of these drugs were advantageous.

I sent Heather home with a specific protocol to support her cycles. This regime included cycled Estriol and Progesterone as well as some supportive supplements.

Heather was diligent at monitoring her cycles and was pregnant for the first time in her life three months later.

Tim and Heather welcomed a daughter and a few years later had a son too.

Samuel and Kendra

I met Samuel and Kendra both age 30 when they visited family here in Illinois. Samuel's sister and husband were established patients and had come to see me in years prior and conceived naturally, they urged her brother and his wife to consult with me too.

I always start by taking a very thorough medical and gynecological history. While Kendra answered my questions, I started to realize that I would have a challenge on my hands.

Due to intense menstrual pain, I learned that she had been taking the oral contraceptive for 15 years. Upon discontinuing the pill, she had noticed that her menstrual cycle was very short. She noted 2 days of thicker reddish/brown bleeding and low pelvic pain.

Her recent past included visits to 2 different reproductive endocrinology practices. She had her infertility evaluations with both clinics to determine that she is in premature ovarian failure. Both antral follicle counts yielded 1-3 follicles for both ovaries. Generally, less than 4 antral follicles represent an extremely low count with no or very poor response to ovarian stimulation expected.

As a fertility specialist I look at lab work and this typically gives a decent picture to accompany the fertility challenge. Kendra's newest blood work was drawn on her cycle day 3. AMH (anti-Mullerian hormone) was undetectable and her FSH (follicle stimulating hormone) was 33. These lab values correlate with her diagnosis of ovarian failure.

Both of the fertility clinics that the couple consulted with advised the couple that they needed to proceed with an egg donor.

Neither Samuel nor Kendra was willing to accept that they needed a donor just yet. Instead, fertility clinic number 2 allowed Kendra to try a medicated cycle to see how she stimulated. The couple and the RE had hoped for one decent sized follicle so they could trigger an ovulation with HCG and time intercourse. Gonal-F (FSH) 300iu was prescribed to be injected each day. She went in for frequent ultrasounds to check for progress and each time there was nothing. No dominant follicle. After 14 days of the maximum dose the clinic discontinued the Gonal-F and told Kendra to allow for her next menses to start.

The couple left feeling hopeless.

After our consult I laid my plan out for them. My plan was to get one more set of cycle day 3 labs and a new AMH. I also wanted to cycle her on bio-identical hormones exactly as her own body would. As we discussed previously, for cases such as these I use high dose DHEA and Pregnenolone. We also needed to get started on utilizing the protocols of the Shared Journey Fertility program. They agreed and came back 2 weeks later to commence.

Kendra reached out 2 weeks after they returned home to let me know that no egg donor was needed and that she had a positive pregnancy test. The couple welcomed a son via an uneventful pregnancy and vaginal birth.

In Conclusion

I f you're trying to have a baby, whether it's your first pregnancy or you want to grow your family, whether you have explained or unexplained infertility issues, know that you have more options than you think.

It's becoming more and more difficult for me to sit back and stay silent about the fertility medicine industry. There is a lot of revenue to be made. I've heard over and over that upon an initial visit to an REI a woman is told in a very positive tone: "let's make a baby" or "we'll get you pregnant." The medical industry is not above profiteering. This, in my opinion, is the ultimate sales tactic, playing on the very delicate feelings of couples that have not been able to conceive on their own. Be cautious. Know your stuff. Since you've come this far, I know that you're already interested in your alternative. As spokesperson of all Merciér Therapists, know we are all standing by. We are midwives, holistic doctors, and healers. We are here to help you and to advocate for your health and safety. We will do whatever we can to aid you on this tumultuous journey, to help you conceive a child in the gentlest way possible. As we have discussed, there are some instances where medical intervention such as various medications or IVF are unavoidable, but together we will see if you're a candidate for a smoother approach. One that keeps you in the driver's seat.

I have been in your shoes. I have sat in front of many REIs as a patient and heard these words ring throughout the room like I'd just been given a free pass to drop the reigns and dutifully follow instructions as they guide me to my baby. These medical professionals are good people with good intentions. They are also fully aware of the stats and the static failure rates from year to year. I have always said there is a time and place for IVF and it is being way overused for nearly all women who walk into a reproductive endocrinology office.

Typically, a less invasive plan such as Clomid or Femara would be tried first. Many women do use these types of cycles and fail because both drugs decrease estradiol production making the vaginal environment hostile to sperm. Many times, this is not explained to their patients. Estradiol is necessary to ensure quality fertile mucous, a robust thick endometrium, and healthy follicle. Plus, there is a higher rate of multiples if the woman does conceive, which must be taken into account when growing your family.

If you do choose to use either of those drugs mentioned above, it is imperative to couple with an intrauterine insemination thus bypassing the hostile vaginal environment.

Insurance wants you to do the less costly cycle first. When you fail three then you are moved up to the bigger guns which is IVF. The numbers are only slightly better.

Most concerning to me are the medical professionals that know absolutely nothing about my practice yet try to steer women away from Merciér Therapy. The tactic is to say that Merciér Therapy doesn't work, and it has no scientific basis. We do not have hefty budgets from big pharma or a large academic institution; therefore a large-scale study is impossible. I know with great certainty that my work yields amazing results, and all without the use of the possibility of harmful or risky medical treatments. In short, there is zero risk in consulting with a Mercier Therapy professional. We are here for you, on your clock, and will work tirelessly to help get you your baby as naturally as possible.

It is my job to guide couples to make a good, sound decision for themselves. I don't say that I have the answer for every case. I don't say that "I'm going to get you pregnant." I don't say that my therapy is always best, really it depends on your situation, but we can find that out with certainty. I don't say that I'll unblock your tubes. I don't say not to work with the medical professional of your choice. I don't say not to do IVF.

The camp that will say all or most of these things is medical professionals because most of them do believe that their way is the best way.

I fully believe that we can work together to provide a better outcome. The division is clear though. I've experienced it time and time again. Reproductive Medicine is a 6.6-billion-dollar industry and these clinics put a lot of merit toward their bottom line. People tend to praise and defend what worked for them.

In 2013, the CDC estimated that 6% of married women in the US, aged between 15 and 44 years, will have issues with infertility. If IVF brought you a baby then IVF is the hero. If Clomid brought you a baby then Clomid is the hero. If you used IUI then IUI is the hero.

How about the naturally and gently conceived pregnancy?

You are the hero for honoring your own body. You are the hero for giving yourself a chance. In the case of very few medically necessary issues some women and men will need intervention. Again, I am not against the medically indicated assisted cycle. However, please look for yourself at the stats on IVF on *SART.org*.

The Society for Assisted Reproductive Technology (SART) collects data from participating clinics in the US. The data is then put into a cumulative sum to give overall national outcomes.

Know that SART is always two years behind in their data collection, but it at least gives an idea as to what you are getting into. I started working in the medical reproductive world in 1994. The stats have not changed that much over the last 25 years. Many of the drugs have evolved but the numbers remain as proof. More potent drugs have been added too, but some of those are so new that there is no way long term health effects can be determined. The data is not abundant.

IVF is taking the process of making an embryo outside of the body; therefore the baby will be created by the hand of another human. There are many factors such as these to consider. What will you do with extra embryos? Freeze them and transfer them at another time? Will you donate them to another couple? How about this… would you donate them to science and allow for stem cell research?

Many of you may not share my moral objections, but I suspect many others of you will.

This is all very hefty stuff to consider, but like I always say, I am here to help.

Please call me or another practicing Mercier provider in your area. We are here to tell you that your body is not broken. That you are not powerless. That making a baby the natural way is not necessarily impossible.

I mean it when I say, Expect a miracle. Miracles do happen every day. I have been witness to several of them day after day, month after month and year after year. The avalanche of positive pregnancy tests is enough to keep me going, but the joy, the relief, and the hope I see on each and every one of my new patients is everything.

Good luck to you and may God bless you on your journey.

Thank You

My endearing thanks to all of the women that have trusted me to care for them on their fertility journey. A deep and heartfelt sense of gratitude to my family, friends, and students for believing in Mercier Therapy and standing next to me as I finished this project. Last but not least, I thank Catherine Borders for editing my pages into an eloquent masterpiece and to Christan Hunsbedt for her beautiful illustrations throughout this book. Ladies, it takes a village and I love you both dearly.

Get in Touch

I wrote this book with the intention of assisting couples to a gentler conception. Please share my work with those who suffer. I would like to change the way we view infertility from a medicalized industry to more of a partnered and conscious approach.

I am thankful that you took the time to read my book and encourage you to follow me on social media and my websites.

For information on professional training in Mercier Therapy:

MERCIÉR THERAPY
professional training

WWW.MERCIERTHERAPY.COM

For information on my clinical practice and
the Shared Journey Fertility program:

EXPECT A *miracle*

WWW.EXPECTAMIRACLE.LIFE

Thank you!

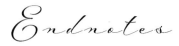

Endnotes

1 My emphasis.

2 Statement given by Saoirse and Conor Walsh.

3 The latter phase of the menstrual cycle or the earlier phase of the estrous cycle. It begins with the formation of the corpus luteum and ends in either pregnancy or luteolysis.

4 The mucous membrane lining the uterus, which thickens during the menstrual cycle in preparation for possible implantation of an embryo.

5 Keep in mind that an optimal endometrial thickness is above 9mm, menotropins can make this much thicker.

6 You can watch their video story on ExpectAMiracle.life.

7 Any of a group of hormones secreted by the pituitary which stimulate the activity of the gonads.

8 JA. Collins JA; M. Bustillo; RD. Visscher; LD. Lawrence. "An estimate of the cost of in vitro fertilization services in the United States in 1995." *Fertility and Sterility*. September 1995.

9 Robin Herman. "Baby-Making in a Test Tube." *The Washington Post*. July 1993.

10 SART.org.

11 Dilation and curettage (D&C) is a procedure to remove tissue from inside your uterus. Doctors perform dilation and curettage to diagnose and treat certain uterine conditions — such as heavy bleeding — or to clear the uterine lining after a miscarriage or abortion.

12 A sonohysterogram is a test in which saline is pushed through the endometrial cavity to examine and make certain that there is no pathology such as polyps or masses present.

13 A fluid filled pouch, and is fairly common post surgery.

14 Her name has been changed to protect her identity.

15 A prosthetic device inserted into the vagina to reduce the protrusion of pelvic structures into the vagina and can be a great option other than surgery.

16 From .2% in her twenties to 5% in her forties.

17 Seifer DB, Baker VL, Leader B. *Age-specific serum anti-Müllerian hormone values for 17,120 women presenting to fertility centers within the United States.* Fertility and Sterility. Reproductive Endocrinology. February 2011.

18 A. Wiser; O. Gonen; Y. Ghetler; T. Shavit; A. Berkovitz; A. Shulman. "Addition of dehydroepiandrosterone (DHEA) for poor-responder patients before and during IVF treatment improves the pregnancy rate: A randomized prospective study." *Human Reproduction*, Volume 25, Issue 10, October 2010.

19 FM. Fusi; M. Ferrario; C. Bosisio; M. Arnoldi; L. Zanga. "DHEA supplementation positively affects spontaneous pregnancies in women with diminished ovarian function." *Gynecol Endocrinol.* October 2013.

20 Regelson W, Colman C. *The Superhormone Promise.* Simon & Schuster. New York, 1997.

21 The first day being the day that menstruation begins.

22 Hashimoto's is an autoimmune thyroid disease in which thyroid antibodies attack otherwise healthy thyroid cells.

23 Synthroid is synthetic T4 (hence its name); it's supposed to convert to T3 which is the active thyroid hormone.

24 N. Kumar, AK Singh. "Trends of male factor infertility, an important cause of infertility: A review of literature." *Journal of Human Reproductive Sciences.* October 2015.

25 Lupron is a hormone therapy. It is classified as an "LHRH agonist."

26 Neil Osterweil. "IVF Linked to Slight Increase in Risk of Some Cancers." *British Medical Journal.* July 2018.

27 N Agarwal, A Subramanian. "Endometriosis - morphology, clinical presentations and molecular pathology." *Journal of Laboratory Physicians.* January 2010.

28 No authors listed. "Revised American Society for Reproductive Medicine classification of endometriosis: 1996." *Fertility and Sterility.* May 1997.

29 Thomas W. Hilgers, MD. *Blinders: The Destructive, Downstream Impact of Contraception, Abortion, and IVF.* Beaufort Books. 2019.

30 Intrauterine Insemination (IUI) is a fertility treatment that involves placing sperm inside a woman's uterus to facilitate fertilization. The goal of IUI is to increase the number of sperm that reach the fallopian tubes and subsequently increase the chance of fertilization.

31 A hysterosalpingogram or HSG is an x-ray procedure used to see whether the fallopian tubes are patent (open) and if the inside of the uterus (uterine cavity) is normal.

32 ART includes all fertility treatments in which both eggs and embryos are handled. In general, ART procedures involve surgically removing eggs from a woman's ovaries, combining them with sperm in the laboratory, and returning them to the woman's body, or in some cases, donating them to another woman.

33 T Kjaer; V Albieri; A Jensen; SK Kjaer; C Johansen; SO Dalton. "Divorce or end of cohabitation among Danish women evaluated for fertility problems." *Obstetrics and Gynecology.* January 2014.

34 Used with permission from the National Catholic Register.

35 AMH (anti-mullerian hormone) is a hormone secreted by cells in developing egg sacs (follicles).